Health Care Professionals' Praise for *What Color Is Your Brain?*® *When Caring for Patients: An Easy Approach for Understanding Your Personality Type and Your Patient's Perspective*

This book will help you put the Patient First and enable you to provide excellent patient care! Every healthcare professional should read this book in order to improve patient satisfaction, relationships with their health care team, and improve communication! The charts are a quick reference you can use daily.

Chris Abercrombie, RN, BS, COHN-S, Environmental Health & Safety Manager, OSF Healthcare System, Ministry Services Facilities Management

WCIYB? is a great system and easy to learn! Understanding an individual's personality traits is paramount in being able to effectively manage any communication cycle. As a clinician, it makes me better equipped to understand my patients and shape my communications in a way they can truly "listen," understand, and accept.

Chuck Schulte, PT, ATC, Diamond Physical Therapy

I love all the health care examples and tables for quick and easy access to the Brain Colors. When our patients are not feeling well and are facing medical obstacles, I have a great resource to be able to connect and provide the most therapeutic support possible and create a healing environment. Thank you for all your Brain Color Magic!

Melissa Bryant, RN, BA, Occupational Nurse Case Manager, OSF Saint Francis Medical Center

This book is a "Must Read!" I was re-energized, while reading Sheila Glazov's and Denise Knoblauch's book, which gives you easy to understand tools and methods that you can use immediately. I will be much more effective improving our employee safety culture and managing change by being better equipped to recognize, accept, appreciate, and adjust my approach to the different Brain Color attributes that everyone brings to the table.

Devon Kelly, MS, OTR/L, Injury Prevention Project Manager, Safety Department, OSF Saint Francis Medical Center

I love this book! After reading it, I recognized my full "Brainbow," personality. Now my clients can receive the best care and knowledge that comes from a balanced combination of mind, body, heart, and soul. Sheila's and Denise's knowledge and insight has now given me the opportunity to help my clients and answer their questions in a "Harmonious, Positive, Simple, and Make Sense Way!"

Lisa Margaret Ash, Owner, IT'S NOT FITNESS...IT'S LIFE!, B.S. NASM, ISSA, ACE, Master/Personal Trainer, Nutritional Specialist

Sheila Glazov has dedicated years of study to a better understanding of relationships between people. Her creativity and enthusiasm for this topic is clearly demonstrated in the unique concepts presented in this book. The importance of building rapport with patients in order to gain their trust and confidence is a critical tool in developing good communication, improved clinical outcomes and patient satisfaction.

Randall E. Marcus, MD, Charles H. Herndon Professor a Orthopaedic Surgery, Case Western Reserve University, University

D1602813

Sheila Glazov skillfully captures the essence of personality types in this easy to read, indispensable gem. See yourself in the unforgettable and relatable stories. Use it to gain a deeper understanding of yourself, which will give you the tools you need to connect with and appreciate your patients on so many levels.

Irene Stemler, RN, BSN, Polytrauma Nurse Educator, Edward Hines, Jr. VA Hospital; Author of *Heroic Acts in Humble Shoes: America's Nurses Tell Their Stories*

This inclusive and encouraging book has made neuroanatomy concepts accessible with clear explanations of the different Brain Colors and how they relate to health professionals and patients. The examples and stories make the information personal, interesting, fun, and uplifting. The organization of the chapters makes it all flow together, reminding us of all the Brain Color attributes and how to apply them.

Dr. Jane A. Richards, DC

I highly recommend this book! It should be a standard text in every health care/ medical office, school, and library. This is the best concept for understanding patient care, coworkers, and workplace dynamics. A harmonious staff equates to excellence in patient care. I wish I was aware of the Brain Color concept when I started my career. Now, my mantra is 'Pause, Color, Communicate."

Carter Black, R.PH, Carter Black, LLC, Pharmacist, Health Consultant and Researcher

I urge everyone who works in the healing professions to read this indispensable book! Sheila and Denise present a holistic approach that, as a therapist, has inspired and helped me understand that each of my clients requires a colorful, unique method to achieve wellbeing. As a manager, it has expanded my awareness of the rare gifts that each staff member possesses.

Jane Zamudio, MA, LCPC, CDVP, MIM, ERYT, Associate Director, Turning Point

This book is a must read for all healthcare professionals! It cuts through the minutiae about understanding your patients' perspective, like a surgeon's scalpel! The relationship with patients and co-workers and the no-brainier conflict resolution chapters will be an immense help to me and my office staff.

Dan Follmer, DDS, NorthWest Dental Health and Aesthetics

Currently, the best approach to the patient is patient centered medicine. Knowing the patient's personality allows an understanding of his or her perspective. This color-filled book allows you to open the patient's heart and compassionately treat the patient as a Person.

Bruno Cortis, MD and author of *Heal Your Cancer, Heart & Soul* and *Healing Heart Disease and The Spiritual Heart*

Great approach! Immediately, I was interested in learning the color of my brain and my patients' and co- worker's brains.

Vivian V. Holman, OTR/L, Edward Hines, Jr. VA Hospital

What Color Is Your Brain?® When Caring for Patients

An Easy Approach for Understanding Your
Personality Type and Your Patient's Perspective

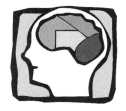

What Color Is Your Brain?®
When Caring for Patients

An Easy Approach for Understanding Your
Personality Type and Your Patient's Perspective

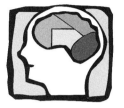

Sheila N. Glazov

Denise Knoblauch, BSN, RN, COHN-S/CM

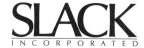

www.Healio.com/books

ISBN: 978-1-61711-834-0

SLACK Incorporated uses a review process to evaluate submitted material. Prior to publication, educators or clinicians provide important feedback on the content that we publish. We welcome feedback on this work.

Published by: SLACK Incorporated

6900 Grove Road

Thorofare, NJ 08086 USA

Telephone: 856-848-1000

Fax: 856-848-6091

www.Healio.com/books

Contact SLACK Incorporated for more information about other books in this field or about the availability of our books from distributors outside the United States.

Library of Congress Cataloging-in-Publication Data

Glazov, Sheila N., 1945-

What color is your brain? : when caring for patients : an easy approach for understanding your personality type and your patient's perspective / Sheila N. Glazov, Denise Knoblauch.

p. ; cm.

Includes index.

ISBN 978-1-61711-834-0 (paperback)

1. Typology (Psychology) 2. Myers-Briggs Type Indicator. 3. Color--Psychological aspects. I. Knoblauch, Denise. II. Title.

[DNLM: 1. Personality Inventory. 2. Personality. 3. Professional-Patient Relations.]

BF698.3.G63 2015

155.2'6402461--dc23

2015008854

For permission to reprint material in another publication, contact SLACK Incorporated. Authorization to photocopy items for internal, personal, or academic use is granted by SLACK Incorporated provided that the appropriate fee is paid directly to Copyright Clearance Center. Prior to photocopying items, please contact the Copyright Clearance Center at 222 Rosewood Drive, Danvers, MA 01923 USA; phone: 978-750-8400; website: www.copyright.com; email: info@copyright.com

Printed in the United States of America.

Last digit is print number: 10   9   8   7   6   5   4   3   2   1

Dedication

To my uncle, Dr. Louis B. Newman, a mechanical engineer, physician, and pioneer and a founding father of physical medicine. As a commander in the United States Navy, Uncle Lou began his medical career by treating injured sailors and Marines during World War II. As a mechanical engineer and a physician, he combined his knowledge and skills to develop rehabilitation practices, therapies, and prosthetics, including a prototype for the Oldsmobile Car Company that put the gas pedal and brake on the steering column for disabled veterans who had lost the use of their legs. Uncle Lou also served as the head of the physical medicine departments in the Oakland, California, and Seattle, Washington naval hospitals. After the war, he became Chief of Physical Medicine and Rehabilitation Services, Hines Veterans Administration Hospital, Maywood, Illinois, and at Lakeside Veterans Administration Hospital, Chicago, Illinois. He also was Professor of Rehabilitation Medicine, Northwestern University, Evanston, Illinois, teaching other physicians and practitioners how to treat veterans and other disabled individuals.

To my father, Alexander I. Newman, a mechanical engineer and president and a co-founder, along with my mother, Sylvia Newman, of Lab-Line Instruments, Inc., which was an industry leader that designed, developed, and manufactured laboratory equipment and instruments for medical and pharmaceutical research and production, clinical health care, academia, and general industry. He was awarded 26 patents for his inventions and laboratory equipment. He was also Building Chairman, Gottlieb Memorial Hospital, which is now part of the Loyola University Health System.

To Sally and Sue, our son, Joshua's, diabetes educator registered nurses, and Libby, Joshua's diabetes educator registered dietitian. Sally, Sue, and Libby were our extraordinary diabetes health care team who offered exceptional patient and family member care, life-saving knowledge, and the crucial skills needed for us to learn to live with the everyday challenges of T1D (type 1 diabetes).

To my cousin, Dr. Alan M. Rogin, a quintessential physician who exemplifies and articulates the distinction between a doctor and a physician in the following statement: "When a student graduates from medical school, he or she is a doctor. During the training period after medical school is the time when a doctor learns how to become a physician. A physician is not only a healer but also is a teacher and guide who offers his or her patients and their families compassion and understanding."

To Dr. David T. Rubin, Professor of Medicine and Co-Director at the University of Chicago Medicine Inflammatory Bowel Disease Center. Dr. Rubin solved my health problems and gave me back my life, gave my husband back his wife, and gave my children back their mother.

To Norman Frankel, PhD, a beloved family friend and business associate of my parents, who thoughtfully introduced me to Dr. David Rubin.

To Carol Childers, CN, LDN, licensed nutritionist and owner of All Ways Healthy Natural Food Center. Carol is passionate about helping people by finding well-researched solutions to their health problems. I regained and maintain my excellent health thanks to Carol's extensive knowledge, compassionate listening skills, dependability, patience, and understanding.

To Chenoa Lorenzo, RYT200, RMT, KRI, owner of Silver Lotus Yoga and my yoga teacher. Chenoa generously and graciously welcomed me into her friendly yoga community and knowledgeably and passionately taught me the benefits of the yoga technology to maintain my health, balance, and strength—physically, emotionally, and spiritually. Namaste.

Contents

Charts Index

Acknowledgments

The **What Color Is Your Brain?**® approach encourages people to recognize and acknowledge their diverse Brain Color attributes and abilities. In this section, I have the privilege and pleasure of acknowledging each individual who shared their Brain Colors and "Praiseworthy Gifts" with me.

My Orange Brain loves a challenge. However, my Blue Brain found this section of the book the most challenging. It was difficult to put into words how much I appreciate my husband, children, grandchildren, family members, friends, colleagues, and clients. I am thankful for their generosity, and I value their copious Brain Color attributes and abilities, which helped to make *What Color Is Your Brain?*® *When Caring for Patients: An Easy Approach for Understanding Your Personality Type and Your Patient's Perspective* a reality!

My Yellow Brain organized each person according to how I thought his or her Brain Color assisted me, which is not necessarily how they see themselves. To be fair, my Green Brain listed everyone's name in alphabetical order.

"Brainbow" Coauthor

My gratitude to my health care professional coauthor and friend, Denise Knoblauch, for her Yellow Brain professionalism, Blue Brain friendship, Green Brain health care knowledge, and Orange Brain sense of humor and fun! I am honored and delighted that Denise agreed to be the coauthor of this book.

"Brainbow" Forward Contributor

My gratitude to Barbara J. Edlund, PhD, ANP-BC, for her Yellow Brain accuracy, Blue Brain thoughtfulness, Green Brain health care expertise, and Orange Brain enthusiasm! I am thrilled and privileged that Barbara agreed to write the foreword of this book.

"Brainbow" Vignette Contributors

"Thank you" to all of the following 31 vignette contributors:

Cathy Cassara, Carole Childers, Jill Cook, Brett Corkran, Teri Elliott-Burke, Michael Epstein, Donna Feldman, Thomas Garcia,

Deb Gauldin, Marylyn R. Harris, Randy Horning, Raymond J. Kayal, Jr., Denise Knoblauch, MaryAnne Kolker, Siri LeBaron, J. Stephen Lindsey, Elaine Long, Maureen Manning-Rosenfeld, Jewel Manzay, Marvin Marshall, Nancy Maruyama, Laura R. Palgon, Clint C. Parram, Matthew L. Primack, Carolyn Roark, Alan Rogin, Virginia Schoenfeld, Ellen Sherman, Donna Tremblay, Sharon Weinstein, and Kristine E. Yung, who entrusted me with their health care stories.

Yellow Brainers

Association of Occupational Health Professionals in Healthcare (AOHP) Executive Board members and Judy Lyle and Anne Wiest of Kāmo Management Services (AOHP's management firm), the Illinois Hospital Association, and Elaine Long.

Blue Brainers

Jill Chambers, Linda Feldman, Kelly Glazov, Doug Gustafson, Raymond Hinkle, Erinn Hughes, Debbie James, RN, and Michael Peterson.

Green Brainers

Gordon Alper, Cater Black, Norman Frankel, PhD (of blessed memory), Dr. Kathrine Kamholz and staff, Raymond Kayal, Jr., Jeff Lewis, and Chenoa Lorenzo, and Silver Lotus Yoga, and Dr. David Rubin

"Brainbow" Publishing Team

To John Bond, the Chief Content Officer at SLACK Incorporated, and my friend, for his Orange Brain enthusiasm for another **What Color Is Your Brain?**® grand publishing adventure.

To Betti Bandura, SLACK project editor and April Billick, SLACK managing editor, for their Yellow Brain editing skills.

To Michelle Gatt, SLACK Vice President/Marketing, for her Yellow Brain "spot on" marketing skills.

"Brainbow" Family and Friends

To my husband, Jordan, for his copious and generous "Praise-worthy Gifts": Yellow Brain "Rependability," Blue Brain AMLF&E, Green Brain critiques, and Orange Brain fun book selling!

To my children and grandchildren for their "Brainbow" of love and blessings!

To Michelle Bracken, my dearest friend, for her Blue Brain encouragement whenever I am "Wet Paint" or "Bright Paint"!

To Doris Shriebman, my dear friend, for her Orange enthusiastic cheerleading and introduction to John Bond, Chief Content Officer, SLACK Incorporated, in 2005. Thank you, "FD!"

"Brainbow" Readers

To my readers, thank you for purchasing my book. Ten percent of the royalties from the sale of *What Color Is Your Brain?® When Caring for Patients: An Easy Approach for Understanding Your Personality Type and Your Patient's Perspective* will be allocated to the Juvenile Diabetes Research Foundation to find a cure and help the children, adults, and their families who live with the never-ending challenges of type 1 diabetes.

About the Author

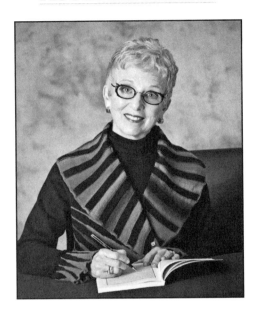

Sheila N. Glazov is an award-winning author, internationally known personality expert, passionate educator, and professional speaker. Sheila's programs and books help individuals decrease the conflict and increase the harmony, collaboration, and effective communications in their homes, workplaces, schools, and communities.

Sheila has appeared on CNN, NBC, ABC, FOX, LIFETIME and WGN-TV. She has been interviewed on Internet programs and radio stations throughout the United States and in Brazil, and featured in the Wall Street Journal, Chicago Tribune, Chicago Sun Times, Daily Herald, and PRAVDA newspapers, iG (largest Brazilian Internet portal), Happy Women (Portuguese magazine), Selling Power, HR, Women's World, Chicago Parent, Seventeen, and Enterprising Women magazines, and the Discover Card and Quill Corporation national customer newsletters. Today's Chicago Woman newspaper selected Sheila as one of "100 Women Making a Difference."

Her innovative style has won Sheila praise for her **What Color Is Your Brain?**® (**WCIYB?**) Programs in conference rooms and classrooms in the United States and around the world. Encouraging adults and children to recognize and respect the best in themselves and others is the essence of her programs and books.

Sheila's programs offer practical and applicable concepts from her popular **What Color Is Your Brain?**® books. During a **WCIYB?** Program, individuals learn to utilize their own "Instant Personality Decoder" to recognize and value their personal perspective and to accept others' viewpoints, improve their job performances, communicate more effectively, resolve conflicts quickly, build healthier relationships, and create harmonious relationships in their professional and personal lives. Adults and children discover their Brain Colors and learn communication skills that go beyond their workplaces and schools, similar to multiplication tables—people never forget!

Sheila's has also authored:

1. **What Color Is Your Brain?**® ***A Fun and Fascinating Approach to Understanding Yourself and Others*** is the original quick and easy personality profile that helps adults and children quickly understand the differences in their personalities. **What Color Is Your Brain?**® has been translated into Portuguese and traditional Chinese.

2. ***Princess Shayna's Invisible Visible Gift*** is an exquisitely illustrated and engaging children's chapter book adaptation of Sheila's book, **What Color Is Your Brain?**® ***Princess Shayna's Invisible Visible Gift*** has been adapted into two musical productions.

3. ***The Teacher's Activity Guide for "Princess Shayna's Invisible Visible Gift"*** is a teacher's resource to apply Princess Shayna's valuable lessons in the classroom.

4. ***Purr-fect Pals: A Kid, A Cat & Diabetes*** is a picture/activity/resource book designed to offer comfort, education, and encouragement to children and their families who live with the challenges of Type 1 diabetes (T1D) and Type 2 diabetes (T2D). Sheila allocates 100% of the royalties from the sale of ***Purr-fect Pals: A Kid, A Cat & Diabetes*** to the Juvenile Diabetes Research Foundation (JDRF).

Sheila allocates 10% of the royalties from the sale of all of her other books to the Juvenile JDRF. Sheila is honored to be a member of the Board of Chancellors, South Jersey Chapter of JDRF. Sheila has first-hand knowledge and experience with the numerous challenges that living with diabetes creates. Sheila's elder son was diagnosed with T1D in 1985, when he was fifteen years old, and her father (of blessed memory) had T2D.

Sheila earned her Bachelor of Science degree in education from the Ohio State University. Sheila has a degree in Creative Leadership from Disney University and is a graduate of the Creative Problem Solving Institute and the McNellis Creative Planning Institute. She has taught 3rd grade and high school English as a Second Language. Sheila has been an adjunct faculty member of William Rainey Harper College and a guest instructor at DePaul, Penn State, and Northwood Universities.

Sheila has been a member of the Professional Speakers of Illinois, the National Speakers Association, the National Speakers Association of Illinois, the Society of Children's Book Writers and Illustrators, the Midwest Writers Association, the National Association for Self-Esteem, the Governors' Commission on the Status of Women in Illinois, Women In Management, Women in Networking, the Women's Task Force for Congresswoman Melissa Bean, and a board member of many community organizations.

Sheila lives in the Chicagoland area with her husband, Jordan.

For more information about Sheila's **What Color Is Your Brain?**® Professional Development Programs and School Programs and her books, please visit http://www.SheilaGlazov.com.

About the Coauthor

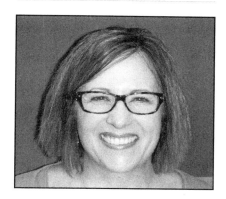

Denise Knoblauch, BSN, RN, COHN-S/CM, is a nationally known health care expert on occupational health nursing. She has spent the past 24 years caring for health care workers. Her patients are hospital employees.

Denise has been employed in the health care field for more than 33 years. She earned an Associate's Degree in nursing from Illinois Valley Community College, Oglesby, Illinois, and received her Bachelor of Science in Nursing from Bradley University. Peoria, Illinois. She has a certificate as a Six Sigma green belt. She is a Certified Occupational Health Nurse Specialist/Case Manager by the American Board of Occupational Health Nurses (ABOHN), a certified hearing conservationist, and a guest lecturer at Illinois State University.

Denise met Sheila Glazov at a **WCIYB?** workshop for occupational health nurses in 2007, and they have been speaking fluent Brain Color since that time. Denise engaged Sheila as a keynote speaker for the national Association of Occupational Health Professionals in Healthcare (AOHP) when Denise was the national conference chair. Denise uses and shares the Brain Color approach and terminology in her personal and professional life on a daily basis, which aids her in adapting communication and accepting of others.

Denise has spent the past 24 years striving to make the workplace safer for health care workers. She has been an active member in all her professional nursing associations. She co-founded her local

AOHP chapter to develop a local networking opportunity for other occupational/employee health nurses. She quickly became a leader at the AOHP chapter level, serving as Vice President, which led to opportunities to serve as a leader at the national level, and she spent 16 years serving as AOHP Executive Secretary, Vice President, President, and President Emeritus. Denise currently serves as the AOHP Continuing Education Co-Chair and the Getting Started on the Road Co-Chair at the national level. She is also leading a team to develop Beyond Getting Starting education for the AOHP members.

Denise has served as The Joint Commission liaison representative for AOHP and was the inaugural AOHP representative on The Joint Commission Nursing Advisory Council.

Denise has mentored numerous occupational health professionals who were new to the field of nursing. She currently serves on the ABOHN and is the Case Manager Chairwoman. Denise has also given professional presentations at the AOHP and the American Association of Occupational Health Nurses (AAOHN) national conferences, AOHP state meetings, and AAOHN regional meetings and presented national webinars for ABOHN regarding obtaining certification as an occupational health nurse.

Denise has participated in the National Institute for Occupational Safety and Health (NIOSH) Public Meeting for the proposed NIOSH Health and Safety Practices Survey of Healthcare Workers. She also served as the occupational health nursing representative for the NIOSH industrial hygiene occupational health committee.

Denise has served on the Department of Homeland Security Infection Prevention and Control Target Capabilities Committee. She had been instrumental in developing the case manager positions at her previous employer. She also was selected as one of inaugural lead green belts in the ambulatory care division, assisting departments in improving health outcomes and functioned as a team leader for projects at OSF Saint Francis Medical Center, Peoria, Illinois.

For 18 years, Denise functioned in a variety of nursing roles in the Occupational Health Department, OSF Saint Francis Medical Center, Peoria, Illinois. Prior to her employment at OSF Saint

Francis Medical Center, Denise was employed at St. Mary's Hospital, Streator, Illinois, for 14 years, working in pediatrics, general medical, home health, employee health, and infection control and prevention nursing roles.

She worked as a telephonic case manager for Erie Insurance Group. Denise admits to being a **Green Brainer** and is amazed that she took a job in which she spends her day on the phone!

She currently works as Executive Director of American Board of Occupational Health Nurses (ABOHN)

Health Care Stories Contributors

Cathy Cassara, CRN, BSN, CHPN, Journey Care, Palliative Services, Hospice, and Hope

Carole Childers, CN, LDN, Licensed Nutritionist; Owner of All Ways Healthy Natural Food Center

Jill Cook, RN, CDE, Renown Diabetes Center, Reno, Nevada

Brett Corkran, BS, MHA, Bon Secours Health System

Teri Elliot-Burke, PT, MHS, BCB-PMD, Co-owner of Women's Physical Therapy Institute

Michael Epstein, MD, Former Chief Operating Officer, Beth Israel Deaconess Medical Center

Donna Feldman, Mother of a child who is a cancer survivor

Thomas Garcia, RRT, RCP (Retired), Northwestern Hospital Medical Center

Deb Gauldin, RN, Professional speaker, humorist, and author, specializing in health care morale and women's well-being

Marylyn R. Harris, RN, MSN, MBA, President, Harrland Healthcare Consulting, LLC

Randy Horning, DC, Owner, Absolute Wellness and Rehab

Raymond J. Kayal, Jr., Esq., Chief Executive Officer and Present, Newslink Group, LLC

Denise Knoblauch, BSN, RN, COHN-S/CM, Executive Director of American Board of Occupational Health Nurses (ABOHN)

MaryAnne Kolker, RN, DN (Retired), New York University Medical Center

Siri LeBaron, MA, Owner of Radiant Lion Yoga

J. Stephen Lindsey, FACHE, Author; Ivy Ventures, LLC, Outpatient Growth Solutions

Elaine Long, FACHE, RYT, CAP, Soul Be It

Maureen Manning-Rosenfeld, MS, LCPC, CDVP, CPAIP, Director of Client Services, Community Crisis Center, Elgin, Illinois

Jewel Manzay, BS, National Sales Manager, Rittenhouse Book Distributors

Marvin Marshall, EdD, Discipline and Parenting Without Stress

Nancy Maruyama, RN, BSN, Executive Director of Education and Outreach, SIDS of Illinois, Inc.

Laura R. Palgon, MEd, Daughter and mother

Clint C. Parram, MPH, Senior Director, Illinois Risk Management Services, An Affiliate Corporation of the Illinois Hospital Association

Matthew L. Primack, PT, DPT, MBA, Vice President of Business Development and Clinical Institutes at Advocate Condell Medical Center

Carolyn Roark, RN, Nurse in a primary care medical office

Alan Rogin, MD, FACS (Retired), Associated Urologists SC

Virginia Schoenfeld, PhD, BCC, Founder of the B.R.E.A.T.H Center

Ellen Sherman, PhD, LMFT, LMHC, The Counseling Resource

Donna Tremblay, BS, MBA, Patient

Sharon Weinstein, MS, RN, CRNI, FACW, FAAN, Author, speaker, Chief Wellness Officer of SMW Group, LCC, and Founder of Core Consulting Group, LLC, and the Integrative Health Forum

Kristine E. Yung, OTR/L, Clinic Director of The Pediatric Place

Preface

After attending my first **What Color Is Your Brain?**® (WCIYB?) workshop with Sheila Glazov in 2007, I was hooked and began speaking Brain Color. It was so easy to relate to the concept, and it helped me to understand work and personal relationships. It was like a light bulb clicking on when I identified my brain color. I was National Conference Chair for the Association for Occupational Health Professionals in Healthcare at that time, and I quickly booked Sheila as our keynote speaker. I wanted our members to have fun while learning to collaborate with others. In true **Green Brain** fashion, I could not imagine anyone not embracing this concept and believed that everyone must learn their brain color.

My relationship with Sheila continued, and our frequent conversations led Sheila to think about another version of **WCIYB?** for health care professionals. She would listen to my stories of what was happening in health care and about all the stresses that health care professionals face while caring for their patients. Hence, this book evolved.

This book will be a quick, easy read for the busy health care professionals who have many demands on their time. Every health care professional is challenged to provide exceptional patient care with the many demands placed on them. My focus has been on employee safety and health, so safety stories are included in the book. You must take care of yourself so you can take care of your patients. Your safety and health impacts your patients.

Please recognize that knowing your patient's Brain Color will help you better relate during the stressful, fast paced events that occur during your shift. Reading this book will help you to assess your environment for Brain Color clues, while interacting with your coworkers, patients, and supervisors. You will see and hear the clues all around you. I hope that as you read each chapter, you will think of the Brain Color stories that have occurred during your career. Health care professionals tell great stories. Now you can include Brain Color connections to make your stories relatable.

Reading this book will give you AH HA! moments as you recognize your patients' Brain Colors and why the interaction was successful or not successful. You will learn ways to improve and enhance each patient's experience while finding ways to decrease the stress in your professional and personal life.

—*Denise Knoblauch, BSN, RN, COHN-S/CM*

Foreword

In their fascinating book, *What Color Is Your Brain?® When Caring for Patients: An Easy Approach for Understanding Your Personality Type and Your Patient's Perspective*, Glazov and Knoblauch provide an invaluable resource for health care professionals to discover and understand themselves, as well as others.

Each of us has strengths and idiosyncrasies that challenge our every day relationships as we try to communicate and interact with patients, colleagues, and other individuals. The authors help us, through the "Brain Quiz" exercises, to gain insight into our own personality type's strengths and perspectives and how one can understand, and thus value and appreciate, the differences in others.

Just like a gemstone, we each have many facets. Although we may exhibit a predominant Brain Color in our interactions with others, the authors encourage us to think more broadly in a "**Brainbow**" of colors to appreciate the contrasting and complementary Brain Colors. Similar to looking through a kaleidoscope, we see an object or situation from many different perspectives. It is this ability that is essential for health care professionals to cultivate to establish effective connections and, ultimately, relationships with patients, coworkers, members of management, and others.

It is this ability that enables health care professionals to modify their approach to educating a patient who thinks very differently than they do. It also is this ability that enables a health care professional to approach administrators with a specific plan to improve care delivery that reflects the key aspects important to and characteristic of the administrator's way of thinking.

The use of numerous anecdotal stories from the many contributors of this book further demonstates the importance of understanding oneself and others, establishing a connection as the basis for relationships, and learning to listen and speak fluently with those of a different Brain Color. The authors note that learning to blend Brain Colors in this way reduces conflict and increases harmony in one's professional life.

A truly insightful, engaging, and an easy read, this book is a "gift" to all health professionals who want to become much more effective in their personal and professional lives.

Thank you for this gift—a grateful **Blue Brain**!

Barbara J. Edlund, PhD, ANP-BC
Professor, Doctoral Program
College of Nursing
Medical University of South Carolina
Charleston, South Carolina

Introduction

Have you wondered why some of your patients are a song in your heart and others are pain in the neck? You will wonder no longer after you read *What Color Is Your Brain?*® *(WCIYB?) When Caring for Patients: An Easy Approach for Understanding Your Personality Type and Your Patient's Perspective*. You will immediately benefit from this effective and easy approach for understanding your personality type and your patient's perspective, which simplifies the complex nature of the adults' and children's personalities with which you interact in your health care workplace.

You are about to learn how to determine and understand your Brain Color personality. This new knowledge will help you increase compatibility with your patients and their advocates, coworkers, and health care management and agencies representatives and improve relationships with your family members and friends.

Over the past 20 years, I have compiled copious **WCIYB?** facts from preparing and facilitating my **WCIYB?** Programs and researching new data about each Brain Color's behavior. I am also honored that 26 consummate health care professionals and individuals generously shared their experiences throughout the book. Their anecdotal stories are strategically placed to complement and enhance the Brain Color information in each chapter. I am confident that the authenticity of each story will offer you inspiration and insights.

You will find the **WCIYB?** concepts fresh, compelling, fascinating, and fun. You will learn quick and simple answers to what makes people tick! **WCIYB?** will also help you to:

1. Understand and value your personality type

2. Recognize and appreciate others' point of view

3. Communicate effectively and resolve conflicts quickly

4. Collaboratively and efficiently reduce frustration

5. Keep your energy up and your stress down

6. Decrease the hassles and increase the harmony in your workplace and at home

I assure you that learning **WCIYB?** will be effortless, educational, and enlightening. The practical applications can be implemented immediately. After a **WCIYB?** Health Care Program, one participant told me, "We're always looking for a way to connect, to relate, to get into someone else's head to understand how they're thinking. Colors are easier and a positive way of identifying personality types, and colors don't label anyone in a way that one might find offensive."

The foundation for **WCIYB?** is the Myers-Briggs Type Indicator, or MBTI®, which is a well-respected, self-reporting assessment tool based on Carl Jung's four personality functions: Sensing, Thinking, Intuiting, and Feeling. I believe the MBTI and other personality assessments offer valuable and valid information. However, their use of a series of letters, terms, and symbols are often complicated and challenging to remember, especially in a world of pin numbers, passwords, and cell phone numbers.

During my **WCIYB?** Programs, I encourage participants to think of **WCIYB?** as an "Instant Personality Decoder" that will help them to decipher their unique characteristics and solve the often puzzling attributes and abilities of others who impact their daily thoughts and actions. Individuals quickly and positively respond to **WCIYB?** because the methodology:

- Uses only four colors to identify personality types.
- Does not label people or put them in only one category.
- Is a nonjudgmental, quick, and easy to learn language that helps people to understand an individual's behavior and feelings.
- Creates a colorful bridge that connects a health care professional's workplace, home, and community.

If the title **What Color Is Your Brain?**® piqued your interest, I'm not surprised. We are naturally and socially inquisitive about ourselves and others. The abundance of television and radio programs, social media sites, blogs, websites, and magazines demonstrate and confirm the curiosity and fascination that individuals have about each other's personality talents and traits.

The essence of my books and programs is to help individuals recognize and respect the best in themselves and others. The **WCIYB?**

personality profiles in this book explain why your perspective differs from or is similar to the viewpoints of others. You can determine your Yellow, Blue, Green, or Orange Brain professional personality in Chapter 1 and your personal perspective in Chapter 10. You may also discover that your Health Care Professional Brain Color may be different than your Personal Brain Color.

I encourage you to use **WCIYB?** as a reference book. Keep it on your desk, in your tote bag or briefcase, or even in your lunchroom at work for quick access to easier conflict resolutions, intriguing revelations, and lively conversations. I trust that you will absorb, embrace, and practice what your have learned to make **WCIYB?** an essential part of your life.

If you have any questions, comments, or health care stories you would like to share with me, please contact me at **sheila@sheilaglazov.com** or leave your message on my website contact page **http://www.sheilaglazov.com/contact**. I would be delighted to hear from you.

Brain Color Daily Reminders:

- Acknowledge your Brain Color "Praiseworthy Gifts"
- Enjoy Each Brain Color Adventure
- Celebrate a Healthy and Happy Brainday every day!

SECTION I

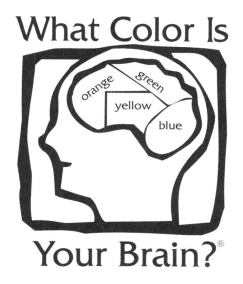

What Color Is Your Brain?®

BRAIN COLOR CONCEPTS

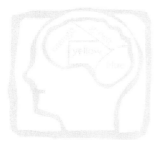

THE HEALTH CARE PROFESSIONAL BRAIN COLOR QUIZ

The **Health Care Professional Brain Color Quiz** is an easy "No Right or Wrong Answer" personality profile that will provide you with an effective tool to analyze your unique characteristics, which will help you recognize your attributes and abilities in the workplace.

MaryAnn Kokler, RN, DN, a senior-staff preadmissions testing nurse, shared with me how she enjoyed utilizing her workplace break time with her coworkers. She said:

> When some of my colleagues and I go on a break, I enjoy sharing the Brain Color information with them. It starts out as a form of relaxation and entertainment. 'What color is my brain? Is this a question and answer quiz?' people ask, as they look over my shoulder at the **What Color Is Your Brain?**® website. I tell them it's a no-brainer. There is no right or wrong color. It is another facet of ourselves. Our personalities reflect the various colors of our brain. Before you know it, they have absorbed the information to deal with others in a more understanding and accepting manner. I think it is kinder to refer to someone by their Brain Color, rather than as an "anal retentive personality!"

The **Health Care Professional Brain Color Quiz** consists of word lists and fill-in-the-blank sentences. The numerical values derived from this process will provide a synopsis of your personality and methodical ranking of your **Professional** Brain Colors.

From *What Color Is Your Brain?® When Caring for Patients: An Easy Approach for Understanding Your Personality Type and Your Patient's Perspective.*
Published by SLACK Incorporated.
Copyright Sheila N. Glazov. http://www.sheilaglazov.com

Nine tips to remember when determining your **Health Care Professional** Brain Color are as follows:

1. Remember to focus on your **Professional** perspective reading the descriptive words and phrases.
2. Your Brain Colors may be different in your health care professional life than in your personal life.
3. You will be able to complete a **Personal Brain Color Quiz** in Chapter 10: *Your Personal Relationship With Family Members and Friends.*
4. Read all the words across the page before you begin to numerically determine their value.
5. If you think two or more words in a row are of equal value, remember your perspective—it is from your **Professional** life. Or, to remind yourself, try the following sentence: In my professional life, I am _____ .
6. You might feel it to be more comfortable and helpful to use "inaccurate" instead of "wrong" and "accurate" instead of "right" when selecting your answers.
7. This is not a "**wanna be**" quiz. It does not determine *who you want to be*, it determines who you *are* at this point of time in your **Professional** life.
8. If you are reading the quiz with another individual, please do not have him or her help you. The purpose of the quiz is for *you* to confirm your own Brain Color. Don't forget—how you see yourself may not be how others see you! According to Rita Carter, author of *Mapping The Mind*, "By the time we are adults, our mental landscapes are so individual that no two of us will see anything in quite the same way."
9. **Enjoy yourself!** The **Health Care Professional Brain Color Quiz** is informative and fun!

Directions

- Read the **four** words and sentences horizontally → across each row on the page.
- Decide which word in each row describes you: *Most* = **4**; *Not as much* = **3**; *Not too much* = **2**; and *Least* = **1**.
- Rank each characteristic in the row across → using 4, 3, 2, and 1 **only once** (i.e., **4** = the **greatest value** and **1** = **least value** to you).
- **Tip:** Read all four choices before numerically ranking your selection.
- After you have completed **all** the rows →, **vertically** add **all** the numbers in **each** of the **four** columns down ↓ to calculate your **TOTALS**.
- Record the **TOTAL** number for your **A, B, C,** and **D** columns in the appropriate **TOTAL** spaces at the bottom of the page.
- If two of your **TOTALS** are numerically equal, this is *not* unusual.

If you add all of your **TOTALS** together, your **TOTAL** numerical ranking should equal **110**.

In Chapter 2: *Recognize Your Professional Strengths and Perspectives*, you will learn details about your personality and how to recognize your Brain Color strengths and perspectives.

The Health Care Profession Brain Color Quiz

A	B	C	D
__ Careful	__ Hospitable	__ Private	__ Confident
__ Meticulous	__ Collaborative	__ Efficient	__ Open-minded
__ Exact	__ Candid	__ Systematic	__ Spontaneous
__ Practical	__ Adaptable	__ Analytical	__ Good-humored
__ Diligent	__ Intuitive	__ Persistent	__ Generous
__ Consistent	__ Authentic	__ Self-sufficient	__ Dynamic
__ Structured	__ Cheerful	__ Cautious	__ Skillful

With patients, I am:

__ Dedicated	__ A good listener	__ Calm	__ Optimistic

With my colleagues, I am:

__ Loyal	__ Helpful	__ Fair-minded	__ Easy going

In my health care workplace, I:

__ Follow rules	__ Am considerate	__ Am realistic	__ Am unbiased

I am most comfortable and thrive in an environment that supports my sense of:

__ Orderliness	__ Cooperation	__ Independence	__Resourcefulness

TOTAL A __   **TOTAL B __**   **TOTAL C __**   **TOTAL D __**

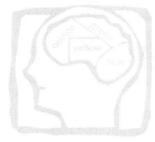

RECOGNIZE YOUR
PROFESSIONAL
STRENGTHS
AND PERSPECTIVES

Wouldn't it be nice to practice?
This fine way of thinking too;
You know something good about me,
I know something good about you!
—Anonymous

You Are a Gem

Someone might describe you as a "gem" because he or she knows something good about you. We often use the word *gem* to describe an individual who is esteemed or valued. To help others understand the **What Color is Your Brain?**® (hereafter referred to as **WCIYB?**) approach, I ask them to think of themselves as multifaceted gemstone-quality people. I have found that people can easily connect to that metaphor visually, emotionally, culturally, and/or historically. Some gemologists believe that gemstones have their own personalities and are valued most for their brilliance of color. Just like a gemstone, we can learn to value our own brilliance and features and understand why we are attracted to the characteristics and radiance of others' personalities.

From *What Color Is Your Brain?*® *When Caring for Patients:*
An Easy Approach for Understanding Your
Personality Type and Your Patient's Perspective.
Published by SLACK Incorporated.
Copyright Sheila N. Glazov. http://www.sheilaglazov.com

Your Best and Brilliant Features

A gemstone is faceted to show off its best features. Over the next few pages, match your **A, B, C, and D TOTALS** from the **Health Care Professional Brain Color Quiz** to each of the four Health Care Professional Brain Color Strengths and Perspectives charts to discover the best and most brilliant features of your personality.

You may find it helpful to read about your Brain Colors according to their numerical sequence. Read first the **A, B, C, or D TOTAL** that ranked the highest, and read last the one you ranked the lowest. You will discover that most of your best and brilliant characteristics are within the Brain Color description you ranked the **highest**.

It is not unusual if two of your **TOTALS** are numerically equal. This indicates similar Strengths and Perspectives in those Brain Colors.

If all your **TOTALS** were closely ranked in a descending order, you will find it easier to shift between your Brain Color attributes and abilities because your Brain Colors are well balanced.

It is normal to recognize a **few** of your characteristics in the other Health Care Professional Brain Color Strengths and Perspectives descriptions. The other Strengths and Perspectives descriptions will also offer insight into other people's best and brilliant features. You will learn more about your Brain Color combinations in Chapter 4: *Understand Your Brain Color Combinations.*

"When we seek to discover the best in others, we somehow bring out the best in ourselves."
—William Arthur Ward

Your Best and Brilliant Perspectives

While you were identifying your Health Care Professional Brain Color Strengths and Perspectives, did you think:

- "This described me to a T."

- "I'm a _____ Brainer and the nurses I work with are mostly _____ Brainers."
- "My department manager is a _____ Brainer."
- "My young patients have lots of _____ in their Brain Color personalities."

Before You Read More

- The term *Brainers* describes or refers to individuals and their Brain Colors.
- For consistency, the sequence of the Brain Colors throughout this book is as follows: Yellow, Blue, Green, and Orange. The Brain Color sequence does not signify a preference for any particular Brain Color or its characteristics. However, note that the left-brain critical thinking and analyzing Yellow and Green Brain Perspectives are on left-hand pages and the right-brain creative thinking and synthesizing Blue and Orange Perspectives are on right-hand pages.

A—MY PROFESSIONAL YELLOW BRAIN STRENGTHS AND PERSPECTIVE

MY ATTITUDE IS: Do it the right way (my way)

I VALUE: Loyalty

IN THE WORKPLACE I AM: Structured

WITH COWORKERS: I am accountable

MY COMMUNICATION STYLE: Direct

WITH PATIENTS: I am dedicated

STRESS: Disorganization

OTHERS SEE ME AS: Controlling

CHANGE: I have to plan for change

I AM RESPECTED FOR MY: Organizational skills

C—MY PROFESSIONAL GREEN BRAIN STRENGTHS AND PERSPECTIVE

MY ATTITUDE IS: Be self-sufficient

I VALUE: Logical problem solving

IN THE WORKPLACE I AM: Efficient

WITH COWORKERS: I like to work alone

MY COMMUNICATION STYLE: Precise

WITH PATIENTS: I am objective

STRESS: Not having the appropriate resources

OTHERS SEE ME AS: Insensitive

CHANGE: I need time to think about change

I AM RESPECTED FOR MY: Technology skills

B—MY PROFESSIONAL BLUE BRAIN STRENGTHS AND PERSPECTIVE

MY ATTITUDE IS: Compassionate

I VALUE: Harmony

IN THE WORKPLACE I AM: Communicative

WITH COWORKERS: I am trustworthy

MY COMMUNICATION STYLE: Inspirational

WITH PATIENTS: I am a good listener

STRESS: Overextending myself

OTHERS SEE ME AS: Too talkative

CHANGE: I intuitively trust my feelings to change

I AM RESPECTED FOR MY: Collaborative skills

D—MY PROFESSIONAL ORANGE BRAIN STRENGTHS AND PERSPECTIVE

MY ATTITUDE IS: Optimistic

I VALUE: Open-mindedness

IN THE WORKPLACE I AM: Quick to respond

WITH COWORKERS: I am energizing

MY COMMUNICATION STYLE: Informal

WITH PATIENTS: I am encouraging

STRESS: Monotony

OTHERS SEE ME AS: Disorganized

CHANGE: I constantly create change

I AM RESPECTED FOR MY: Skills in getting results quickly

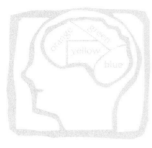

3

APPRECIATE AND ACCEPT OUR DIFFERENCES

"There is a sense of our characters caring for each other and respecting each other. A positive feeling. A positive view of life. That's the key to everything we do."
—Jim Henson, creator of the Muppets

Care, Appreciation, and Respect

The following are eight essential ways that Alan M. Rogin, MD, FACS, a Yellow/Blue Brain physician, cared for, appreciated, and respected his patients and health care colleagues for more than 45 years. His goal was to make every patient feel nurtured, accepted, and supported. We trust you will find Dr. Rogin's list helpful and encouraging:

1. "I believe I delivered on my promises to care for my patients to the best of my ability."

2. "If I thought I could not provide the best care for my patients, I found another physician with the appropriate skills."

3. "My goal was for each individual to feel that I was not just listening to him or her but actually hearing what he or she had to say."

13

4. "I always made it a point to acknowledge a patient's fears, whether he or she expressed them openly or not. I believe that anyone who is referred to a specialist has an element of fear, whether it is a diagnosis they fear hearing or the fact that he or she may be facing a surgical intervention."

5. "Occasionally, a patient would become upset over what he or she considered to be a prolonged waiting time in my office. I always explain that I take as much time that is needed for each individual patient, and, occasionally, that takes longer than expected. I also point out that I am prepared to spend as much time as he or she needs for their appointment."

6. "If I felt a patient was not listening to me or was disrespectful to my staff, and the issue could not be resolved satisfactorily, I would not hesitate to suggest that he or she find another physician."

7. "Over the years, I developed mutually respectful relationships with my colleagues, both in the office and in the hospital. This was especially true in the operating room where, by working closely with the nursing staff, we were able to implement many policies and procedures that directly led to much improved patient care, resulting in better outcomes. To do less was not an option."

8. "One of the great gifts given to me was the opportunity to sit and listen to the stories that my patients from the Greatest Generation shared with me. Although their bodies may have looked increasingly frail on the outside, they were still young and strong on the inside."

I felt I had achieved my goals when after my retirement I received a letter from a long-time patient in which he stated that although the new doctor was doing a good job, *'but he is not Dr. Rogin. You are a great physician and a caring person, and incidentally, thank you for saving my life. Both my wife, Lorraine, and I miss you and wish you good health and God's blessing.'*

A Positive View of Life

The positive sense of an individual's character and self-confidence is influenced by his or her values and feelings of contentment. When you are self-confident, you have the ability to feel acceptance, self-worth, capability, empowerment, respect for yourself and others, and to solve problems effectively.

Your interaction with the other Brain Colors in the health care workplace, at home, and/or in your cultural community influences your positive view of life. Misunderstandings between people often are a result of not appreciating and accepting another individual's unique personality traits.

WCIYB? will help you to:

1. Recognize how other people's personalities affect you
2. Value what is meaningful, relevant, and significant about each personality type
3. Acknowledge and respect the diversity of your patients and the other individuals in your health care workplace

An Explanation, Not an Excuse!

The **WCIYB?** approach does *not* focus on tolerance. Tolerance can be defined as:

1. A fair and objective attitude
2. The act of enduring or putting up with

I think most of us would like others to have a fair and objective attitude toward us but not a sense of tolerance. By definition, this would cause others to endure or just "put up" with us.

The focus of the **WCIYB?** approach is *acceptance* and *appreciation* of yourself and others, and to learn how to recognize and understand the harmonious and hazardous individuals in your professional and personal life.

Please remember that **WCIYB?** is an explanation, not an excuse, for people's inappropriate behavior.

Stimulant and Subliminal Effect

Color is a major stimulant in our lives and profoundly influences our behavior, such as the clothes we wear, the cars we drive, the advertisements we read, or how we respond to other people's behavior and the color of their hair, eyes, and skin. Historical, educational, religious, and/or cultural interpretations influence the environmental conditions that expose us to colors, or the lack of colors. These influences may also have a subliminal effect on us, similar to the effects demonstrated in the following examples:

- You find it easy to comfort the Yellow Brain husband of one of your patients. He reminds of your favorite high school Spanish class teacher.

- Your affectionate Blue Brain mother had red hair. Whenever you see female patients with red hair or if they remind you of your mother, you want to hug them.

- It is challenging for you to relate to the new emergency department physician. He reminds you of your Green Brain grumpy neighbor who always yells at the neighborhood children when they make too much noise and disturb him.

- Two Orange Brain rambunctious little boys come to your occupational therapy class each week. Their behavior reminds you of your younger brothers and the fun you had with them when you were children.

Basic Brain Facts

Some facts about the average human brain are as follows:

- Its size is approximately 400 grams, or 0.88 pounds (or 14 ounces).

- Its weight is between 1.2 to 1.5 kilos, or 3.0 to 3.3 pounds.

- It weighs only 2% of the body's mass.

- It uses 25% of the energy that a body requires to operate per day, which is 500 calories of 2,000 calories required to keep the human brain functioning.
- Its neurons are the functional information processing units of the brain.
- It has approximately 86 billion neurons.

The Yellow Brainers

The **Yellow Brain** section of the **WCIYB?** illustration is the temporal lobe. There is a temporal lobe on both sides of the brain, and it relates to recognizing and processing sounds, emotions, and our ability to remember, understand, and produce speech. If a temporal lobe is injured, an individual's hearing, language, ability to recognize familiar faces, and the processing of sensory information may be affected.

Notice that the Yellow section contains a right angle. **Yellow Brainers** need to be "right." Rules are the foundation of a **Yellow Brainer's** life. They are recognized as left-brain critical thinkers who provide structure and stability in their professional and personal lives. Their punctuation mark is a period because they frequently make declarations.

Historically, ancient Romans and Egyptians saw yellow as the color of their sun gods. Yellow can be mentally stimulating and boost your alertness. Many religions connect yellow to a spiritual path of unity, glory, and a Supreme Being or deity. Yellow also can represent power and wisdom.

The Ayurvedic Science/Medicine and Energy Healing aspects of the third (solar plexus) chakra are the positive use of personal power, control, awareness, and manifestation of personal goals.

Yellow Brainers thrive on the responsibilities of leadership. They select health care professional careers as chief executive officers (CEOs) of health care systems, hospital administrators, admissions clerks, risk managers, dietitians, and security officers. Their professional careers in non-health care fields often include chief operating officers (COOs), event planners, educators, bankers, business managers, and administrators.

Recognizing a **Yellow Brainer's** Behavior: A Yellow Brain department manager of a breast center becomes annoyed with her team members' behavior—the **Blue Brainers** are talking, the **Green Brainers** are looking at their smart phones, and the **Orange Brainers** are looking at the clock.

Yellow Brainers build their self-confidence with behavior that is "as good as gold." A traffic signal represents a Yellow Brainer's "I need to be in control" attitude.

The Blue Brainers

The **Blue Brain** circular section of the **WCIYB?** illustration is the occipital lobe. It is located at the back of the brain and relates to the physical ability to see and receive and process visual information. It also helps an individual to perceive colors and shapes. If the occipital lobe is injured, an individual's vision may become impaired, his or her field of vision may become distorted, and he or she may perceive sizes, colors, and shapes differently.

The occipital lobe symbolizes insightfulness and the attribute to connect with others. **Blue Brainers'** intuition correlates with their right-side brain creative thinking and their "the sky's the limit" perspective. Their punctuation mark is a question mark because they like to ask questions about other people to learn more about them. They often have to ask questions because they were talking and did not hear what was being said.

Historically, the Romans and Greeks attributed the color blue to Venus, the goddess of love. The **Blue Brainers'** perspective is one of love and peace. Blue has been used in studies to relax muscles, lower blood pressure, and was found to calm hyperactive children. In the Buddhist tradition, blue produces peace of mind and equanimity. The Ayurvedic Science/Medicine and Energy Healing aspects of the fifth (throat) chakra are the expression of dreams, finding new connections, sharing, self-expression, and joyful communication of their creative discoveries.

Blue also represents the sky, coolness, and water. All three meanings symbolize a **Blue Brainer's** ability to be in the creative flow. The ancient Greeks believed that blue is the color of truth.

Blue Brainers thrive on being "true blue." They select health care professional careers as nurses, social workers, child life specialists, pediatric nurses and physicians, mammography technicians, hospital volunteer coordinator, and wellness specialists. Their professional careers in non-health care fields often include artists, social workers, musicians, child care providers, and pet care specialists.

Recognizing a **Blue Brainer's** Behavior: A **Green Brain** dietician speaking to a group of diabetes educators says, *"People, listen up, this information is critical."* A **Blue Brainer** responded, *"But I was just being helpful and showing Sylvia an app about fruits and veggies."*

Blue Brainers build their self-confidence on truthfulness, authenticity, and helping others. A light bulb represents a **Blue Brainer's** "I've got a great idea" attitude.

 # The Green Brainers

The **Green Brain** section at the top of the **WCIYB?** illustration is the parietal lobe. The parietal lobe is a mini-computer that integrates sensory information from other parts of the body. It processes cold, hot, pain, touch, which direction is up, and helps us from stumbling into objects. If an individual's parietal lobe is injured, he or she may have trouble locating and recognizing parts of his or her own body.

Green Brainers are proficient problem solvers, avid readers, and adept with computers. They need to be independent and like to work by themselves. Their punctuation mark is a comma because left-brain critical thinkers need to pause and contemplate what they are going to say before they speak. They never want to look or feel incompetent.

Historically, the color green has symbolized growth, tranquility, and freshness. Green can reduce stress and can be calming.

In various cultures, the color green represents hope, long life, and immortality. The Hindu tradition states that green is the color of knowledge, memory, and the ability to see into the future.

The Ayurvedic Science/Medicine and Energy Healing aspects of the fourth (heart) chakra are fresh new growth because the heart is the dispatcher of information, personal consciousness, and expression of feelings through actions not words.

Green Brainers are visionaries who thrive on innovation and select health care professional careers as therapists (physical, occupational, respiratory), surgeons, neonatal nurses, performance improvement specialists, lab technicians, and x-ray technicians. Their professional careers in non-health care fields often include accountants, computer professionals, scientific and medical researchers, engineers, and lawyers.

Recognizing a **Green Brainer's** Behavior: A **Green Brain** x-ray technician has been practicing the AIDET (Acknowledge, Introduce, Duration, Explanation, Thank you) technique but is frustrated and complains to a coworker, saying, "*I am experienced and knowledgeable, but sometimes I comes across as bragging and being a know-it-all. I try to balance everything and not make it sound like I am saying 'and where did you get degree from?' and putting off the patient.*"

Green Brainers build their self-confidence by acquiring and imparting knowledge and solving problems. A "do not disturb" sign represents a **Green Brainer's** "I must to be alone to think" attitude.

 # The Orange Brainers

The **Orange Brain** asymmetrical section of the **WCIYB?** illustration is the frontal lobe, which takes the longest to mature and does not completely develop until an individual is between the ages of 25 and 30 years. This lobe involves impulse control, decision making, selective attention, controlling behavior, and emotions. If an individual's frontal lobe is injured, it may affect how he or she

handles his or her emotions, impulses, selection of appropriate language, and social and sexual behavior.

The frontal lobe shape represents the **Orange Brainers'** fluid
thoughts and actions. **Orange Brainers** appear to be constantly on
the move, both physically and mentally. This movement represents
their ability to create change and be thought of as right-brain creative
thinkers. You have probably guessed the **Orange Brain** punctuation
mark—an exclamation point, of course! They thrive on excitement,
action, adventure, and risk taking.

Historically, according to Chinese tradition, the color orange represents a powerful energy source and stimulator. To the Japanese,
the color orange signifies happiness and love. Buddhist monks wear
orange robes as a symbol of humility.

The Ayurvedic Science/Medicine and Energy Healing aspects of
the second (sacral) chakra are a glow and "pow" of awareness, explo-
ration about an individual's physical attributes and abilities, and
creative forces being utilized for the different facets of an individual's
personality. Orange is a mixture of red and yellow, which symbolizes
excitement, energy, and the glowing flame of a fire. The color orange
is reported to boost the appetite and stimulate communication.

Orange Brainers select health care professions careers as emergency department physicians, nurses, and technicians; emergency
medical technicians, paramedics, recreational therapists, house-
keepers, maintenance workers, cafeteria workers, marketing managers, and hospital fitness/wellness center trainers. Their professional careers in non-health care fields often include firefighters, law
enforcement officers, sports professionals, construction workers, and
sales professionals.

Recognizing a **Orange Brainer's** Behavior: A hospital offered a
health and nutrition event to encourage employees' life style changes.
At the conclusion of a two-mile walk/run, the dietetic interns chuckled and said, "This is the worst parade ever!"

Orange Brainers build their self-confidence by demonstrating
their courage and getting results quickly. A juggler, keeping a variety

of objects or tasks in the air, represents an **Orange Brainer's** "I can do it all" attitude.

It's Not Easy Being Green

When I am conducting a **WCIYB?** program, I ask the participants to stand up, take a stretch from sitting in their chairs, and visually demonstrate their group's Brain Color statistics, which generally represent the adult population of their professional or personal perspective:

> - 35% to 40% Yellow Brainers
> - 35% to 40% Blue Brainers
> - 10% to 15% Green Brainers
> - 10% to 15% Orange Brainers

Generally, the following is representative of a health care workplace:

- Department managers are Yellow Brain responsible organizers.
- Nurses are Blue Brain helpful nurturers.
- Physicians are Green Brain problem solvers.
- Trauma team members are Orange Brain individuals who get results quickly.

However, depending on the composition of the attendees of a **WCIYB?** program, the number of Brain Colors will vary. For example, a program for CEOs, religious leaders, and administrative assistants will have more Yellow Brainers; nurses, day care owners, and elementary school teachers will have more Blue Brainers; medical researchers, physicians, and engineers will have more Green Brainers; and emergency department staff, emergency medical technicians, and sales professionals will have more Orange Brainers.

The previous percentages demonstrate diversity in a group, such as a hospital or community service organization. If the program participants are attorneys, technology managers, or engineers, the largest percentage will be Green Brainers; however, if the participants are not from these careers, the Green Brainers will possibly be the smallest group represented.

In every program, I ask the Green Brainers to raise their hands to visually show their Brain Color. I do not ask them to stand up to visually display their Brain Colors. I am sensitive to Green Brainers' desire to not stand out in a crowd, which is the opposite of other Brain Color participants.

Unlike the enthusiastic Orange Brainers, who jump out of their chairs as if they were cheerleaders, the Green Brainers hesitate, look around for others who did not stand up or raise their hand, and then see their fellow Green Brainers' hands. They might then hesitantly raise their hand to let the other Green Brainers know who they are. That is my cue to bring Jim Henson's celebrated Muppet, Kermit the Frog, stage center. I ask the group, "What does Kermit say?" and a chorus of "It's not easy being green!" echoes through the room.

Yes, it is not easy for the Green Brainers because they are most misunderstood for being pessimistic, instead of being cautiously skeptical. They are not as comfortable demonstrating or communicating their feelings as are the other Brain Colors. Actually, Green Brainers can be more sensitive than the other Brain Colors; they just do not wear their hearts on their sleeves like the Blue Brainers. Yellow Brainers say it is not easy for them because they worry about their responsibilities; Blue Brainers because they become overwhelmed about personal issues; and Orange Brainers because their excitement creates too many activities for them to realistically handle.

"Only the Shadow Knows"

When any of the Brain Colors say "it's not easy," that indicates they are feeling what Carl Jung would describe as "Shadowed"—the subconscious negative, or dark side, of your personality. Historical and cultural symbols of the shadow include snakes (as in the Garden of Eden), dragons, monsters, demons, and the Devil.

If your Comfort Color, which is your dominant Brain Color that represents your personality's strengths and comfort level, is "Shadowed" you may feel boxed in, restricted, stereotyped, labeled, or defined in a way that does not make you feel positive, confident, or trusting about yourself and others.

Notice that the head in the Brain Color logo seems to be pushing out of the box. **WCIYB?** allows you to expand your personality and become more than you appear to be. Observe that the Brain Color head is not precise and that the shadow of the head does not exactly fit into the illustration. These imperfections are a visual metaphor of our personalities: No one likes to be put in a box or feel like they must be perfect.

A **Shadowed Orange Brainer**, who thrives on creative chaos, might find it difficult to understand and work with a **Yellow Brainer**, who thinks the **Orange Brainer** is unreliable, because the **Yellow Brainer** values structure and accountability.

A **Shadowed Green Brainer**, who focuses on the problem and not on the emotion that the problem creates, might find it difficult to understand and work with a **Blue Brainer**, who feels hurt by what he or she feels is the **Green Brainer's** lack of sensitivity.

Comparing Differences

Author Marvin Marshall, EdD, asks a simple question in his *Comparing Yourself With Others* newsletter article:

D o you compare crayons?
Comparing is such a natural activity that we become a victim of its effects. Every time you compare yourself with another and

think lesser of yourself, you fall into the abyss of a useless activity. Your feelings fall with you, and you have gained nothing.

On the other hand, the opposite occurs when you feel better because you think you are better than the other person. Your feelings soar. But to what avail? Does it add to your humanity to know that you are 'better' than someone else?

Think "different"—not better or worse. (This, by the way, is what diversity is all about.)

As youngsters use crayons, they should be taught that, although all are different, they all make contributions. We pick and choose because of the differences, but this does not mean that one is better than the other. Which is a better color: red, blue, purple, green, orange, yellow, etc.?…As the artist uses colors for different purposes, learn from others, but refrain from comparing.…

How Are You Feeling?

Understanding our differences and knowing that individuals can be a silhouette of themselves will help you interpret "I'm not feeling like myself today" from a Brain Color perspective. You will learn more about your Shadowed personality and how it affects conflict and compatibility in Chapter 15: *No-Brainer Conflict Resolution and Creative Problem Solving.*

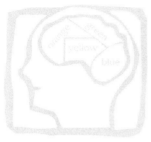

UNDERSTAND YOUR BRAIN COLOR COMBINATIONS

Sir Isaac Newton discovered that when a prism broke up light, it revealed a continuous play of color—a rainbow. By definition, a rainbow is the following:

- A spectrum of brilliant color.
- Highly varied or multifaceted.
- Any multicolored arrangement or display.

Your "Brainbow" Personality

The structure and relationship among the colors in a rainbow is not definitive. The colors harmoniously blend one into the next, just as you will learn to blend your Brain Colors to reduce conflict and increase harmony in your professional life.

You could select one or all of the definitions to describe your Brain Colors, or "Brainbow." In the previous chapters, you gained insight into each personality type's strengths and perspectives and how you can appreciate their differences. Now that you have identified the numerical sequence of your Professional Health Care Brain Colors, you can examine the full range of your "Brainbow" to appreciate the contrasting and complementary Brain Colors.

From *What Color Is Your Brain?® When Caring for Patients:
An Easy Approach for Understanding Your
Personality Type and Your Patient's Perspective.*
Published by SLACK Incorporated.
Copyright Sheila N. Glazov. http://www.sheilaglazov.com

The four Brain Color designators are as follows:

- **Comfort Color**
- **Blending Color**
- **Convertible Color**
- **Clouded Color**

The color you determined to have the highest value on your Professional Brain Color Quiz is your **Comfort Color;** this is your dominant Brain Color. It represents your strengths and comfort level in most situations and demonstrates your **Bright Brain Color Behavior**. The highest possible value for any Brain Color is 44. One of my clients determined that her Comfort Color was Blue. Her B TOTAL of 40 (of a possible value of 44) demonstrates that she glows like a blue neon light bulb! She sees herself as creative and flexible and feels the most comfortable in communicative and cooperative situations.

The color you determined to be the second highest value is your **Blending Color**. Depending on its numerical ranking, it influences your Comfort Color and helps you to easily shift between those two Brain Colors. The D TOTAL of 34 is my client's Orange Blending Color, an indication of her courage and enthusiasm, which influences and encourages her dynamic personality.

The color you determined to be third in value is your **Convertible Color**. It is in the median ranking and can exchange positions with your Blending Color or Clouded Color. One of my client's A TOTAL of 32 is her Yellow Convertible Color. She often feels like the woman in artist James Christensen's painting, *The Responsible Woman*, flying through the air carrying symbols of her home, career, family, friends, and community. The value of 36 of Orange as her Blending Color and value of 32 of Yellow as her Convertible Color demonstrates that she can easily switch back and forth between those two colors to become a resourceful woman.

The color you determined to have the lowest rank is your **Clouded Color**. It often is the spark that ignites conflict with yourself and others, demonstrating **Shadowed Brain Color Behavior**. The Clouded Color designator of another client's personality is her lowest ranking of 11 in the C (Green) TOTAL. She is diligent about using her Green brain instead of her Blue heart. When people make a request of her, she says, "I need time to think about that" before she offers an answer or makes a commitment. She also has learned to be grateful for the Green Brainers in her life. They compensate for her analytical deficiencies and rationally encourage her when her personality is Shadowed.

You can learn more about the concept of Shadowed Colors in Chapter 3: *Appreciate and Accept Our Differences* and in Chapter 15: *No-Brainer Conflict Resolution and Creative Problem Solving.*

Making Harmony Happen

Being aware of your Brain Color combinations will help you avoid conflicts and create more harmony in your professional life within yourself and with others.

Specific colors combine well, whereas others conflict. As you learn more about your Brain Colors, it will become obvious that the Yellow perspective will have more difficulty blending with Orange, as will Green with Blue. Conversely, the Blue perspective will blend easily with the Orange perspective because they are right-brain creative thinkers who find it easy to synthesize their thoughts, and the Yellow perspective with the Green because they are left-brain critical thinkers who find it easy to analyze their thoughts.

You will find it easier to blend your Brain Colors if the numerical sequence of your Brain Colors is equally distributed and numerically balanced. You also will be more adaptable, accepting, and patient with others and yourself. Conversely, if the numerical sequence is unequally distributed and numerically imbalanced, you will find the opposite to be true.

A Comfortable Blending

Your Comfort Color and your Blending Color are your first and second Brain Colors; they have the most influence on your perspective and behavior. Consequently, if your Comfort Color is Yellow and your Blending Color is Orange, you are a Yellow/Orange Brainer. Use this model whenever you blend two Brain Colors. The more your Comfort Color score exceeds your Blending Color score, the more dominant your Comfort Color will be.

Your Comfort Color/Blending Color combination can be complementary or conflicting. As you may have noticed, the Yellow and Orange characteristics are usually opposite each other; likewise, the Blue is opposite Green. As a result, Yellow/Orange Brainers experience conflict because their Yellow sense of responsibility clashes with their Orange desire for fun; the Blue/Green Brainers struggle between their Blue emotions and their Green logic.

Your Brain Colors, or combinations, can influence and benefit other people's Brain Colors, as can theirs influence and benefit yours. A Yellow Brainer can influence a Blue Brainer's decision about his or her medical office. The benefit is that people and ideas thrive because they are working in a collaborative and orderly environment. An Orange Brainer can influence a Green Brainer's indecision about remodeling his or her physical therapy office. The benefit is that recommendations for quality furniture and functional storage units that can be purchased at reasonable prices and installed by a reliable contractor quickly provide the results the Orange Brainer wants.

A Beautiful "Brainbow" Blending Personality

I had the privilege and pleasure of collaborating with Elaine Long, FACHE, RYT, CAP, who was the Leadership Development Consultant at Advocate Condell Medical Center. Elaine is a perfect example of a beautiful "Brainbow" blending of an individual's Brain Color Personality.

Elaine hired me to present **WCIYB?** at an Advocate Condell Medical Center Leadership Development Institute (LDI) program. I was immediately impressed with Elaine's professionalism, knowledge, and attention to details. Elaine designed the program and worked with a diverse group of medical staff members to ensure that we accomplished all the learning objectives and goals.

She always was efficient, responsive, and flexible. Elaine was 100% engaged and invested in the collaborative and creative process to make the LDI program a success. She demonstrated quintessential management skills while organizing and directing the diverse groups.

Elaine demonstrated exceptional communication and team-building skills that were strategic, innovative, and encouraging. Elaine's attributes and abilities definitely made a remarkable and memorable difference for those of us who worked with her and for the attendees at the LDI program, who had a positive and enjoyable experience.

The following are examples of Elaine's "Brainbow" Personality:

- **Yellow Brain:** Preplanning 6 months in advance, incorporating updates, and two rehearsals.
- **Blue Brain:** Collaboration with me and the other speakers.
- **Green Brain:** Strategies and objectives for the event and other speakers.
- **Orange Brain:** A fun "cruise" theme, with decorations in the four Brain Colors, energetic music, and superb prizes.

Know Your Strengths

Before experiential learning conference attendees participated in Low Ropes team-building activities, I taught them the **WCIYB?** methodology. I encouraged them appreciate their differences and to transfer and apply their Brain Color knowledge during the activities. It was fascinating to observe the interaction among the participants, who had not known each other before the conference.

- The **Yellow Brainers** explained the rules and organized the group into smaller teams.

- The **Blue Brainers** encouraged each participant as he or she navigated the course and congratulated him or her when finished.
- The **Green Brainers** evaluated the obstacle risks and developed systems that everyone could utilize to complete the course safely.
- The **Orange Brainers** eagerly demonstrated techniques to nimbly walk the tightrope, quickly negotiate obstacles, and cooperatively pass teammates through a giant rope web.

Knowing the strengths of their Comfort and Blending Colors positively influenced the participants' diverse attributes and abilities, enhanced their self-confidence, and motivated them to work as a team to complete the obstacle course successfully.

"Brainbow" Combinations

The following examples of possible **Comfort**, **Blending**, and/or **Convertible** colors will help you to recognize and value the following "Brainbow" combinations:

 YELLOW "BRAINBOW" COMBINATIONS

- Yellow/Yellow: Dependable/Planner
- Yellow/Blue: Responsible/Nurturer
- Yellow/Green: Prepared/Researcher
- Yellow/Orange: Organized/Negotiator

 BLUE "BRAINBOW" COMBINATIONS

- Blue/Blue: Sensitive/Naturalist
- Blue/Orange: Creative/Improviser
- Blue/Yellow: Affectionate/Caretaker
- Blue/Green: Helpful/Innovator

GREEN "BRAINBOW" COMBINATIONS

- Green/Green: Curious/Inventor
- Green/Yellow: Well-informed/Planner
- Green/Blue: Technical/Trainer
- Green/Orange: Independent/Troubleshooter

 ORANGE "BRAINBOW" COMBINATIONS

- Orange/Orange: Resourceful/Negotiator
- Orange/Blue: Risk taker/Team player
- Orange/Yellow: Fun-loving/Organizer
- Orange/Green: Entrepreneurial/Problem solver

Your "Brainbow" on a Tridge

The combinations of your "Brainbow" personality are significant because your contrasting and complementary Brain Colors can vibrate to create tension, as well as talent. Your "Brainbow" perspective is your reality at work, home, and in your community.

During all of my **WCIYB?** programs, I show a slide of **The Tridge**, which is the formal name of a three-way wooden footbridge spanning the convergence of the Chippewa and Tittabawassee Rivers in Midland, Michigan. For many years, I enjoyed walking across **The Tridge** when I was teaching classes at the Alden B. Dow Center for Creativity and Enterprise and attending the annual conference that the Center hosted for individuals who taught creativity classes at universities and colleges.

My slide demonstrates another basic foundation concept of **WCIYB?**—each individual is like **The Tridge**. Our "Brainbow" personality equally joins and balances our attributes and abilities and allows us to metaphorically travel among our Brain Color perspectives and environments, which include our workplaces, homes, and communities (Figure 4-1).

Figure 4-1. Metaphorical Tridge diagram.

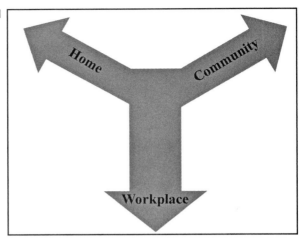

*The sharing of joy,
whether physical, emotional, psychic, or intellectual,
forms a bridge between the sharers,
which can be the basis for understanding much of what is not
shared between them,
and lessens the threat of their difference.*
—Audre Lorde

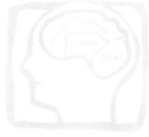

HOW OTHER BRAIN COLORS SEE YOUR BRAIN COLORS

"For what you see and hear depends a good deal on where you are standing:
it also depends on what sort of person you are."
—C.S. Lewis

Brain Color Glasses

How we see another person is similar to a writer's point of view (POV), which is in the perspective of the story or character and how that viewpoint is revealed. To reveal your POV, imagine wearing a pair of Brain Color glasses that are tinted Yellow, Blue, Green, or Orange. However, remember that how you see yourself may not be how others see you because of *their* Brain Color glasses. In specific situations, others' POV might be more significant than how you see yourself.

From *What Color Is Your Brain?® When Caring for Patients:*
An Easy Approach for Understanding Your
Personality Type and Your Patient's Perspective.
Published by SLACK Incorporated.

There Were Three Men

The following poem, written by John Masefield, was a gift from my Yellow/Green Brain friend, Jewel Manzay. I use Jewel's poetry gift in all my programs to demonstrate the significance of how we see ourselves, how we would like to see ourselves from our Brain Color POV, and how others view us from their Brain Color POV.

Three Men
There were three men,
Went down the road
As down the road went he.
The man they saw,
The man he was,
And the man he wanted to be.
—John Masefield

Point of View

Fundamentally, we differ in our values, needs, motivations, wants, and beliefs. **WCIYB?** may help you understand that you cannot change another person. You can change only your POV about them through recognition, acceptance, and appreciation of their strengths and perspectives. However, it is easier to see your POV, as well as someone else's, when you are wearing Brain Color glasses.

Author David Kiersey wrote, "If I do not want what you want, please try not to tell me that my want is wrong. Or if I believe other than you, at least pause before you correct my view."

Black Leather

During my programs, I reinforce the "how others see your Brain Color" concept by asking participants to collaborate with another person and share something about themselves that other people would not know from their appearance or by speaking with them. This is the "true confessions" entertainment segment of the workshop. People have discovered that their medical office manager is a champion horsewoman, their pediatric nurse is a tap dancer, and their operating department doctor is an accomplished fly fisherman.

To the program participants, my physical appearance and conduct conveys that I am a capable and responsible businesswoman. Then, I show a video clip of me and my husband riding on our motorcycle. The video was taken before my hair turned to silver sparkles, and many program attendees do not realize it is me. I know others realize it is me because they watch in disbelief. When the video ends, I disclose, "What you cannot tell by looking at me is...I am a Hog Harley Mama who rides on the back of a 'Bagger' in black leather, and I am a Biker Bubbe!" I make my point and everyone laughs.

Depending on other people's Brain Color perspectives, you might be surprised about how they see you and may understand their positive or negative perception. This was true when my husband and I were on one of our annual motorcycle vacations. We were out riding one morning and decided to stop in a jewelry and gift store that friends told us not to miss. Dressed in our leathers, it was fascinating to observe how deliberately the salespeople ignored us. I decided to conduct a Brain Color experiment, so later that day, we returned to the same store dressed in our conventional vacation clothes.

Several of the same salespeople approached us to ask if we needed any help. "No thank you" I said, "We are just looking." However, we were not looking at the merchandise, we were looking at them. They needed the help. Their perception of how a customer should look cost the store a sale and my customer satisfaction.

The charts starting on page 38 will show you how others positively and negatively see your Brain Colors according to their POV.

—Sheila N. Glazov

How Others See Your Brain Colors—The Yellow Brainer Perspective

Yellow sees Yellow as:	Yellow sees Green as:	Yellow sees Blue as:	Yellow sees Orange as:
Organized	Abstract	Honest	Impulsive
Dependable	To the point	Harmonious	Impatient
Conservative	Problem solver	Spiritual	Fun
Loyal	Intellectual	Genuine	Opportunistic
Predictable	Perfectionist	Devoted	Manipulative
Tenacious	Reserved	Sensitive	Out of control
Traditional	Boring	Compassionate	Manic
Stable	Logical	Sympathetic	Impulsive
Decisive	Smart	Helpful	Creative
Punctual	Independent	Emotional	Disorganized
Responsible	Superior	Authentic	Late
Realistic	Withdrawn	Intuitive	Messy
Firm	Nonsocial	Indecisive	Belligerent
Effective	Condescending	Team player	Active
Caretaker	Thinkers, not doers	Moody	Impractical

From *What Color Is Your Brain® When Caring for Patients: An Easy Approach for Understanding Your Personality Type and Your Patient's Perspective*. Published by SLACK Incorporated. Copyright Sheila N. Glazov. http://www.sheilaglazov.com

How Others See Your Brain Colors—The Blue Brainer Perspective

Blue sees Blue as:

Creative
Emotional
Intuitive
Nurturing
Communicative
Helpful
Moody
Compassionate
Pleaser
Sympathetic
Empathetic
Harmonious
Trusting
Flexible
Romantic

Blue sees Yellow as:

Organized
Anal retentive
Not creative
Structured
Fighters for their point
Not liking disruption
Rigid
Respectful
Uncompromising
Self-righteous
Goal oriented
Loyal
Neatniks
Orderly
Domineering

Blue sees Green as:

Way too intelligent
Intimidating
Academic
No common sense
No people skills
Too analytical
Inflexible
Smart
Intense
Focused
Cold
Uncaring
Independent
Isolated
Uncommunicative

Blue sees Orange as:

Fly by seat of pants
Courageous
Good sense of humor
Disorganized
Not detail oriented
Just wants results
Fun
Annoying
Adventurous
Carefree
Adaptable
Enthusiastic
Competitive
Expedient
Resourceful

From *What Color Is Your Brain?® When Caring for Patients: An Easy Approach for Understanding Your Personality Type and Your Patient's Perspective.* Published by SLACK Incorporated. Copyright Sheila N. Glazov. http://www.sheilaglazov.com

How Others See Your Brain Colors—The Green Brainer Perspective

Green sees Green as:	Green sees Yellow as:	Green sees Blue as:	Green sees Orange as:
Productive	Bureaucratic	Emotional	Impulsive
Logical	Controlling	Caring	Courageous
Innovative	Orderly	Empathetic	Cavalier
Knowledgeable	Organized	Relationship focused	Spontaneous
Superior intellect	Task oriented	Concerned	Intuitive
Curious	Computational	Warm	Fun
Fair minded	Rigid	Smothering	Unreliable
Objective	Impeccable	Mothering	Illogical
Selective	Dependable	Valuable	Valueless
Precise	Traditional	Helpful	Spontaneous
Visionary	Know-it-alls	Too talkative	Inconsistent
Rational	Self-righteous	Idealistic	Self-absorbed
Reasonable	Historians	Touchy-feely	Change agent
Cool, calm, and collected	Planners	Fighters for a cause	Idea generator
Efficient	Prompt	Creative	Impetuous

From *What Color Is Your Brain?® When Caring for Patients: An Easy Approach for Understanding Your Personality Type and Your Patient's Perspective*. Published by SLACK Incorporated. Copyright Sheila N. Glazov. http://www.sheilaglazov.com

How Others See Your Brain Colors—The Orange Brainer Perspective

Orange sees Orange as:	Orange sees Yellow as:	Orange sees Blue as:	Orange sees Green as:
Decisive	Controlling	Friendly	Nerds
Capable	Organized	Sensitive	Fact finders
Smart	Scheduling	Romantic	Eggheads
Fast moving	Structured	Creative	Geeks
Influential	Opinionated	Poetic	Number crunchers
Not liking routine	Stubborn	Caring	Studious
Fun loving	Inflexible	Lovers	Slow moving
Hands-on learner	Jailers	Helpful	Analyzers
Skillful	Self-righteous	Cooperative	Plodding
Good negotiator	Frustrating	Loving	Intellectual
Problem solver	Judgmental	Understating	Dull
Proficient	Too scared	Compassionate	Dry
Athletic	Boring	Listeners	Insensitive
Results provider	Stringent	Nurturers	Ice cold
Risk taker	Safe	Intuitive	Condescending

From *What Color Is Your Brain?® When Caring for Patients: An Easy Approach for Understanding Your Personality Type and Your Patient's Perspective.* Published by SLACK Incorporated. Copyright Sheila N. Glazov. http://www.sheilaglazov.com

"Sweetest"

It is easy to recognize your own admirable personality traits, but it is often difficult and uncomfortable to recognize the annoying ones. However, if you utilize the **WCIYB?** approach, I think you will be more comfortable with yourself and more accepting of others.

One morning, the meeting planner for the American Academy of Pediatrics' staff team-building program introduced me to the attendees. The Orange/Blue Brainer concluded her introduction with "and Sheila is one of the sweetest people I know!"

I responded to the "sweetest" comment with a grimace that made everyone laugh. As I stepped up to the podium, I added, "Your colleague and I did not plan this, but this is a perfect example of why you are here this morning. She sees me as sweet, but I would never describe myself as sweet … kind or caring, but *not* sweet!"

The meeting planner used her Orange/Blue brain to be spontaneous and helpful about introducing me. Because of my Blue/Orange Perspective, I was not offended. I knew she was being creative with my introduction. In fact, I was delighted that she contributed her personal feelings to the group because it gave me the opportunity to comment on how her behavior transferred and applied to the program.

If Ms. Orange were Yellow or Green, she would not have ad libbed. She would have respected my request and read the introduction precisely as I had written it. We could not have created a better introduction or interaction with the group if we had planned it.

Point of View Differences

I encourage you to pause before you tell someone he or she is wrong or attempt to correct his or her POV, and consider the POV that Glenn Frank, American editor and educator, offers in his poem, *The Difference.*

When the other fellow acts that way,
He is ugly;
When you do, it's nerves.
When the other fellow is set in his ways,
He is obstinate;
When you do, it's firmness.
When the other fellow takes his time,
He is dead slow;
When you do, you are deliberate.
When the other fellow treats someone especially well,
He is toadying;
When you do, it's tact.
When the other fellow finds fault,
He's cranky;
When you do, you are discriminating.
When the other fellow says what he thinks,
He is spiteful;
When you do, you are frank.

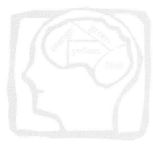

THRIVE IN
IDEAL AND
SAFE CONDITIONS

"Health care is a dangerous profession, even though controls are available to reduce unsafe conditions and control hazards. The incidence rate for work-related, nonfatal injuries and illnesses in health care is 1.3 times more than the average worker in the United States."
—Denise Knoblauch, BSN, RN, COHN-S/CM

As an Occupational Health Nurse, the following is my Top 10 List for an Ideal and Safe Employee Health Care Environment:

1. The ideal health care environment would have all the technology available to prevent and reduce the risk of injuries.

2. The staff would have time to use such protection and have easy access to prevention measures while providing safe, efficient, and compassionate care.

3. The patients would be easy to care for and would listen to staff.

4. The staff would be able to easily approach patients without fear of being hit or attacked.

5. The managers would have time to investigate employee injuries.

6. The mangers should have an effective root cause analysis in place so that all risks to employees could be discovered and ultimately eliminated.

From *What Color Is Your Brain?® When Caring for Patients: An Easy Approach for Understanding Your Personality Type and Your Patient's Perspective.* Published by SLACK Incorporated.

7. The staff would be compliant with wearing personal protective equipment and completing medical surveillance exams on time.

8. The staff would perform exceptional hand hygiene, thereby reducing hospital-acquired infections.

9. All employee injuries would be eliminated.

10. Workers' compensation costs would be eliminated so that hospitals would have less overhead expenses and could provide care to all patients, regardless of ability to pay.

—Denise Knoblauch, BSN, RN, COHN-S/CM

Ideal Brain Color Workplaces

 ### *YELLOW BRAINERS' IDEAL WORKPLACE*

- Long-term planning
- Recognition for a job well done
- Manuals and procedures
- Well-trained support staff
- Definitive job description and responsibilities

 ### *BLUE BRAINERS' IDEAL WORKPLACE*

- Interaction among employees
- Shared decision making
- Relaxed company policies
- Flexible work schedule
- Personalized work space

 ### *GREEN BRAINERS' IDEAL WORKPLACE*

- State-of-the-art equipment
- Research resources
- Independent work schedules
- Opportunities to use problem-solving skills
- Innovative systems

ORANGE BRAINERS' IDEAL WORKPLACE

- Immediate monetary rewards for achieving results
- A variety of challenges
- Locations for relaxation and/or physical recreation
- No schedules or meetings
- Freedom to take action

Is It Nature or Nurture?

By now, you might be wondering how nature and nurture affect an individual's personality. Is your personality determined by your environment or gene pool? My fundamental nature versus nurture belief is this: the conditions of an environment or setting have a significant effect on the nurturing of an individual's natural temperament. I agree with the premise that an individual's personality is a combination of both the person's natural characteristics (nature) and how he or she is raised (nurture) and how he or she is encouraged or discouraged, which determine personality traits and behavior.

We are living in a time of rapid change, which significantly impacts your Brain Colors. Sometimes the conditions of your surroundings or another person's behavior can cause you to feel uncomfortable or unsafe.

A specific environment will nurture the natural traits of an individual. A **Green Brainer** and a **Yellow Brainer** will not be as comfortable or productive in an unscheduled brainstorming session as will a **Blue Brainer** or an **Orange Brainer**.

Opposite Brain Color settings, as long as the environment is trustworthy, can nurture your natural attributes and abilities. Trustworthiness is the ability to accept others and their contributions, to support, recognize, and affirm others' strengths and capabilities, and exhibit cooperative and honest intention. People thrive when their attributes and abilities are acknowledged!

You are capable of changing your environment and making conscious decisions to nurture yourself. Some Brain Colors adapt to change easier than others. In Chapter 17: *You Can Change Your Brain Color* you will learn more about what prompts you to change.

Helen's "Brainbow" Patient Environment

by Denise Knoblauch, BSN, RN, COHN-S/CM

Helen was a 3-year-old girl who was born with esophageal and tracheal defects. She had been confined to a hospital her entire life, as she was unable to eat and required assistance to breath. Her family had to visit her every day in the neonatal intensive care unit in Korea. Her family longed to find a cure for her problems and take her home. A Blue Brain nurse from my hospital was in Korea on a teaching assignment and met Helen.

This Blue Brain nurse contacted a Blue Brain pediatric surgeon to try to find help for Helen and her family. The surgeon did some research and found another surgeon in Sweden who had done research on cell development, which could help Helen. Unfortunately, his hospital in Sweden did not have the funds available to perform the necessary surgery.

The concerned Blue Brain surgeon used his Yellow Brain dedication to not give up easily. He approached the medical center's administration to bring Helen and her family to our facility for the ground-breaking surgery. It took a committed team of "Brainbow" staff to provide the care and technology for Helen and her family.

The development of a Blue Brain-based compassionate hospital unit, which included family-centered patient rooms in the children's hospital and in the pediatric intensive care unit, offered Helen's family their first opportunity to stay together at all times during Helen's hospitalization.

The Green Brain research surgeon cultivated the cells to repair Helen's trachea. It took each surgeon's Brain Color attributes to perform the complicated surgery, which involved three major organ systems. Helen survived the complicated ground-breaking surgery.

Listening to Helen's "Brainbow" health care team tell her story was extraordinary. The Blue Brain surgeon told Helen's story so eloquently and tenderly. The Green Brain research surgeon cautiously relayed his part of the miracle. Another surgeon used his Yellow Brain to discuss all of the detailed technical aspects of Helen's surgery. The Orange Brain staff members shared how they thought of fun ways to help Helen experience all the "firsts" in her life. While at our hospital, Helen was able to taste her first lollipop!

Sadly, a few weeks after the ground-breaking surgery, Helen began to lose her battle. However, the whole hospital rallied around Helen and her family.

Although I was not directly involved with her care, Helen's story touched me and demonstrated how all the Brain Colors can work together to become a "Brainbow", and resulted in offering a young patient and her family an exceptional experience and patient care. Although the outcome was not what was expected, my coworkers and I rejoiced that Helen and her family were able to experience a stronger Blue Brain family bond within the confines of our hospital.

Be Watchful

To enhance your awareness of the ideal conditions in which your Brain Color thrives, be watchful to visually recognize the unique characteristics that reveal an individual's Brain Color. The following descriptions of Brain Color workspaces may be helpful in recognizing such unique characteristics:

 Yellow Brain Clean-Up Coaches

Their workspace and/or desk are clear of any clutter. Awards are hung sequentially and straight on the wall. It is so neat that it looks as if no one works there.

 Blue Brain Cozy Collectors

Their workspace and/or desk looks like someone's family room. It is accessorized with comfortable furnishings, flowers, memorabilia, and family or pet photos.

 Green Brain Selective Savers

Their workspace and/or desk is large enough to keep all their projects within reaching distance. They will have the latest technology, a collection of books on the floor or on shelves, and their diplomas displayed on the wall.

 Orange Brain Clutter Champions

Their workplace and/or desk and floor space resembles a display of stalagmites, but they know exactly what is in each of their piles. They do not spend time organizing their office or desk because it is a waste of time.

"All I Want Is A Place Somewhere … Oh, Wouldn't It Be Loverly?"

by Anonymous Hospice Nurse

As a nurse working in hospice, I have traveled from home to home and was able to, in a ritualistic sort of way, step out of my car and close the door on the concerns of my prior visits and personal life. Doing this allowed me to enter the next home with a clear Blue Brain. This is far more difficult to do in the hospital environment. I would find myself rushing from room to room to assess patients, provide care, give medications, answer call lights, and try to make the time to listen and address patients' concerns. Finding a free moment from rushing between rooms to center oneself to allow for a therapeutic interaction would, I think, require a more deliberate and conscious effort.

The hospital environment not only affects a patient's well-being, their perception of stress, and their ability to heal well, but it also impacts nursing and hospital staff. The hospital environment is full of stressful encounters, as well as noise from monitors, alarms, and overhead paging systems that impact the staff's ability to do their jobs well and with intention. It is essential for health care workers to have a place where they can decompress and return to their patients in a healthier state of mind. Recognizing this need, I have begun to work on a proposal for a meditation, or tranquility, room, where staff could go to take time away from the overstimulating environment to regain their centeredness.

It is important, in my mind, that the room be dedicated to personnel only, separate from families and patients, to allow meditation time to be uninterrupted and directed inward; a space that is nurturing to the human spirit, where staff can remove their shoes, empty their pockets, and put evidence of work aside, so that they may enter the room unencumbered.

A room such as the one proposed would allow staff members to clear their minds and open their hearts, which would ultimately improve the quality of their work, increase patient safety and care, and improve clinical outcomes.

Not Playing It Safe!

Denise Knoblauch, BSN, RN, COHN-S/CM, shared the following anecdotal stories from her experience as an occupational health professional at a large community hospital. Each story is a precarious reminder about the consequences of "not playing it safe!"

- The **Yellow Brain** employee would call the Occupational Safety and Health Administration (OSHA) to complain about what he or she perceived to be an unsafe condition that had not been corrected. The employee might also complain to his or her manager that someone else's negligence and/or not following the rules had caused him or her to incur an injury. The Yellow Brain employee needed to be right and point out which individuals were not following *the* rules.

- The **Blue Brain** nurse in the Neuro ICU (neurological intensive care unit) had to give a patient two injections. She had to remember which medicine was in each syringe so she could properly document medication administration. It was a very busy weekend evening shift, with many demands on her time. She gave injection #1 and set down the used syringe without activating its safety mechanism. After giving the injection #2, she stuck herself, while picking up the used syringes.

  ▷ Her Blue Brain had been distracted, was in a hurry, and absentmindedly failed to follow protocol of using the appropriate and available technology.

- The **Green Brain** pregnant x-ray technician became enraged when she entered a room to take a patient to the x-ray department and discovered the critical fact that the patient should have been in isolation for possible tuberculosis. This exposed her and her fetus unnecessarily.

▷ When she confronted the **Orange Brain** nurse who was in charge of the patient and who failed to post the necessary signage at the entrance of the room, the nurse said, "I was going to get around to it."

• The **Orange Brain** emergency department technician was working in a code situation. She drew the patient's blood but had to walk across the room to dispose of the needle in the sharps disposal box. A coworker was crossing the room at the same time. The two technicians ran into each other and the Orange Brain technician was stuck with the used needle.

▷ The **Green Brain** worker's compensation staff person wondered why the sharps disposal box couldn't be put closer to the place of use and why the staff person was using a nonsafety needle device.

▷ The **Yellow Brain** worker's compensation staff person wanted to go the unit and remove all the nonsafety needle devices and change the ordering system so that no one could order nonsafe needles in the future.

Remain Alert for Gifts!

Remain alert to the ideal and safe conditions in which your Brain Colors will thrive. Your awareness is crucial for building relationships with your patients and colleagues, for solving problems, and making healthy decisions in your health care workplace.

A mantra I created for myself many years ago, one I have shared with others and want to share with you is:

> If you are aware, the gifts will be there. Some of the gifts may be metaphorically wrapped in beautiful paper and decorated with colorful ribbons and others maybe covered in ugly worn and torn wrapping paper and frayed and faded ribbons. What really matters is not the gift's appearance but how you decide to receive or welcome the gift into your life.

SECTION I: BRAIN COLOR CONCEPTS SUMMARY

Brain Color Perspective	Yellow Brainers	Blue Brainers	Green Brainers	Orange Brainers
My attitude	Do it the right way	Compassionate	Be self-sufficient	Optimistic
I value	Loyalty	Harmony	Logical problem solving	Open mindedness
My communication style	Direct	Inspirational	Precise	Informal
Brain lobes	Temporal	Occipital	Parietal	Frontal
Change	I plan for it	I intuitively trust my feelings about it	I think about it	I constantly create it
I am respected for	My organizational skills	My collaborative skills	My technology skills	My skills to get results
Build my self-confidence	With "good as gold" behavior	By helping others	By imparting knowledge	By demonstrating courage
How others see my Brain Color personality	Realistic, orderly, controlling, rigid, accountable	Nurturing, caring, moody, smothering, trustworthy	Visionary, efficient, insensitive, intense, intelligent	Skillful, decisive, unreliable, unstable, adventurous
Ideal workplace conditions	Procedures and trained staff	Relaxed policies and personalized space	Independence and innovative systems	Challenges and no meetings
In the workplace, I am...	A clean-up coach	A cozy collector	A selective saver	A clutter champion

From *What Color Is Your Brain?® When Caring for Patients: An Easy Approach for Understanding Your Personality Type and Your Patient's Perspective.* Published by SLACK Incorporated. Copyright Sheila N. Glazov. http://www.sheilaglazov.com

SECTION II

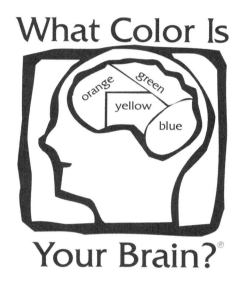

What Color Is Your Brain?®

BRAIN COLOR PROFESSIONAL AND PERSONAL CONNECTIONS

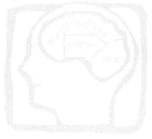

YOUR RELATIONSHIP WITH PATIENTS

No Respect or Compliance

by Donna Tremblay

As a Green Brain patient, I arrived precisely at 2:00 PM for an appointment with my new and highly recommended internist because I was suffering from vertigo. When I looked around the narrow room for a seat, eight of the 10 chairs were occupied, and the big-screen TV was blaring with an obnoxious game show.

I quickly spotted the office receptionist, who was sitting behind her desk discussing the contestants of the TV game show with the two other staff members, who were also focused on the craziness on the TV screen.

As I approached the desk, the receptionist said, "Hi, what is your name?" in a voice level louder than the television. I felt like I was in front of a machine gun firing squad as the receptionist shot the following questions at me: "Do your have your insurance information? Is this is your correct billing address? Is this your date of birth? Why are you here to see the doctor today?"

Each time I was questioned, I replied in my normal composed tone of voice. However, the receptionist had to shout, "Speak up. I can't hear you over the raucous volume of the television."

From *What Color Is Your Brain?*® *When Caring for Patients:
An Easy Approach for Understanding Your
Personality Type and Your Patient's Perspective.*
Published by SLACK Incorporated.
Copyright Sheila N. Glazov. http://www.sheilaglazov.com

After answering the receptionist's barrage of questions, I took the only seat remaining in the reception room, which was directly under the blaring big-screen TV. As I attempted to get comfortable, I felt as if seven pairs of eyes, which knew the private details of my life, were fixated on me and not on the ridiculous game show. If I closed my eyes, I would have thought I was waiting in a car repair shop, where the mechanic needed to know what was wrong with my car, not a doctor's office.

I was relieved when it was my turn to see the doctor and he was able to give me a prescription that cured my vertigo. However, I never returned to the doctor's office because my patient privacy had not been respected, and the HIPAA [Health Insurance Portability and Accountability Act] privacy rules to protect my medical records and other personal health information were not complied with!

Patients' Brain Colors

When dealing with patients, do you feel like a Yellow Brain prison warden, a Blue Brain doting grandparent, a Green Brain science teacher, or an Orange Brain summer camp counselor? It is difficult to pinpoint just one personality and behavior because of the information you may not have about your patient and/or the patient's circumstances.

The information in this chapter will examine how to connect with adult and pediatric patients to effectively interact with them and build relationships to meet their needs according to their Brain Colors.

Adult Patients' Brain Colors

Connecting with adult patients and their advocates to build a trustworthy relationship requires the following attributes and abilities:

 ### FOR YELLOW BRAIN ADULT PATIENTS
- Communicate clear instructions.
- Provide a health care plan.

- Explain details about their care.
- Offer realistic expectations.
- Respect their decisions.

FOR BLUE BRAIN ADULT PATIENTS

- Offer encouragement.
- Be an attentive listener.
- Validate their feelings.
- Be quiet and let them talk about their feelings.
- Don't be afraid of their emotions.

FOR GREEN BRAIN ADULT PATIENTS

- Keep the situation objective and unemotional.
- Understand that they can be very sensitive.
- Do not get frustrated when they do not give you an immediate answer. They need time to process.
- Ask precise "Yes" or "No" questions.
- Provide explanations about medical procedures and listen to their perspectives.

FOR ORANGE BRAIN ADULT PATIENTS

- Respect their feelings about losing their sense of freedom.
- Do not come across as "bossy."
- Help them to understand the end result.
- Explain the consequences.
- Keep the conversations easy going.

A Patient's Friend

by Tom Garcia, RRT, RCP

As a hospital respiratory care practitioner, I had a special relationship with one particular patient. She became a quadriplegic as the result of an incident in which she was an innocent bystander.

Her name was "Iris," and I was immediately captured by her vibrant personality and optimism in the face of such a catastrophe. Iris had a Green/Orange brain attitude and a beautiful smile. She was the kind of patient who made health care a rewarding and satisfying career. Iris always had a positive outlook, which put my Blue/Yellow Brain into overdrive. I always enjoyed being assigned to treat her. I visited Iris whenever she was admitted, even if I wasn't assigned to treat her. She would tell other respiratory care practitioners to let me know she was in the hospital, just so we could visit and catch up. We had an authentic and warm Blue Brain relationship. I would give her a hug and kiss her forehead whenever I saw her, even when we were passing each other in the hospital halls.

On one of Iris' many admissions, she became withdrawn and unresponsive and went into a trance-like state not uncommon of patients in her condition. I went to see her and did my best to get through to my dear friend, drawing on all the color-filled lobes of my brain. Iris did not blink. My heart ached to see her in such a distressing condition. My Blue Brain took her condition very personal. I felt like I had failed her as a professional and as a friend.

The next time Iris was admitted to the hospital, I had an opportunity to tell her how it hurt me to see her so ill during her last hospital admission. Even though Iris couldn't remember the incident, she told me how sorry she was.

Thinking about Iris always reminds why it is so rewarding to take care of a patient who is as thoughtful, positive, and pleasant as Iris.

Pediatric Patients' Parents/ Guardians/Advocates

When working with pediatric patients, you need to be aware of their age and treat them in an age-appropriate manner, understand their developmental differences, be considerate of their "very real" concerns, and acknowledge their need for security, compassion, and comfort, which are influenced by their Brain Colors.

It also is critical to respect the child's parents, guardians, or advocates. Physical therapist, Matthew L. Primack, PT, DPT, MBA, created the term, "Thought Partner," which is a perfect description of the person or persons who are parenting, caretaking, or advocating for a pediatric patient, who may not be capable or mature enough to process information about his or her care or condition. A "Thought Partner" is an adult who is able to responsibly and logically think, respond, and make decisions about the child's care and condition.

You can also encourage Thought Partners to keep a journal and record critical information that they and their child's health care team can use as a resource when making decisions about the child's health care and condition.

For Yellow Brain Pediatric Patients (and Their Parents/Guardians/Advocates)

1. Offer them detailed information about their care.
2. Give them structured and step-by-step directions to take care of themselves.
3. Respect their age and level of understanding.
4. Understand their feelings of insecurity.
5. Allow them to talk about their illness without interrupting with your opinion.

For Blue Brain Pediatric Patients (and Their Parents/Guardians/Advocates)

1. Validate their feelings.
2. Listen attentively and sincerely.
3. Reassure them that you and your colleagues are available to help them.
4. Let them cry if they need to.
5. Hug them, if appropriate.

For Green Brain Pediatric Patients (and Their Parents/Guardians/Advocates)

1. Respect their privacy.
2. Do not touch them without asking their permission first.
3. Do not tell them they are "wrong."

4. Do not treat them as a "baby."

5. Provide explanations about their care and the reasons why it is being done.

 ## For Orange Brain Pediatric Patients (and Their Parents/Guardians/Advocates)

1. Use activities and stories to explain information.

2. Reassure them that you are opened minded about their concerns.

3. During conversations, get to the point quickly.

4. Use play to help them feel more comfortable.

5. Foster their need for self-expression.

My Baby and the Wicked Witch of the West

by Donna Feldman

I was a Blue Brain mother attempting to comfort my 6-month-old daughter, who had just been diagnosed with neuroblastoma. We were in the children's hospital to begin her chemotherapy and steroid treatments. However, my baby was not tolerating the steroid medicine, which she also had to use for treatment of the cancer, and it was making her extremely fussy and unmanageable. My Blue Brain was emotionally upset and frightened with thoughts about my baby dying.

I knew my little one was scheduled for more tests, and I wanted her to get some much needed rest. I hoped that holding my daughter would help to calm and comfort her and myself. Finally, my baby settled down, fell asleep, and I was able to put my daughter in the crib for a nap.

My baby and I were both exhausted. No sooner had I begun to relax, knowing my daughter was resting peacefully, when a stern-looking nurse appeared at the end of my daughter's crib. Without introducing herself, the Yellow Brain nurse barked, "I have to take her vitals, temperature, and measure her urine."

I attempted to calmly and protectively explain that my daughter had just fallen asleep and I did not want the nurse to waken her.

The nurse flung a mean scowl at me and replied, "This is my job, I have to do this. This is my job, it has to be done." I felt like the nurse had transformed into the Wicked Witch of the West from the *Wizard of Oz* movie. This Neon Yellow Brain nurse acted as if she were wearing a blindfold and could not see my emotional fatigue and distress about my daughter. My Blue Brain mother's intuition felt as if I could read the nurse's thoughts that were racing through her Yellow Brain: "What is wrong with this mother? Why is she so frightened about her baby? Well, too bad for you, lady. I am going wake up your baby and do my job!"

And she did!

Addendum: Donna's daughter is now a healthy, joyful, intelligent, and talented young woman!

Patients' Family Members

Adults' and pediatric patients' family members play a significant role in your patients' health care. I have heard patients' family members complain about chasing a heath care professional down the hall to get an update about their loved one and being told that they do not need to know, or not having their questions answered, or being treated as if they are invisible.

Remember Matthew L. Primack's "Thought Partner" term that was mentioned earlier in the chapter? It is a perfect description of patients' family members who are caretaking or advocating for a loved one who is not capable of processing information about his or her care or condition. A patient's Thought Partner will be able to responsibly think, respond, and make decisions about his or her loved one's care and condition. The following information will help you to respond appropriately to a patient's family member Thought Partner:

For Pediatric Patients' Yellow Brain Family Members

1. Be direct.
2. No sugar coating.
3. Be respectful.
4. Give medical reports and updates promptly.
5. Be on time for meetings.

 ### *For Pediatric Patients' Blue Brain Family Members*

1. Choose your words wisely because they are sensitive.
2. Be patient.
3. Try to be flexible about their concerns and requests.
4. Recognize that they may be overly emotional.
5. Offer a hug, if appropriate.

 ### *For Pediatric Patients' Green Brain Family Members*

1. Respect their family privacy.
2. Know that they are not forthcoming with information.
3. Use short notes, texts, or e-mail to communicate health updates.
4. Give them time to process information before making a decision.
5. Offer them appropriate health care resources.

 ### *For Pediatric Patients' Orange Brain Family Members*

1. Speak to them in a familial and informal manner.
2. Whenever possible, share appropriate notes your have taken about the patient.

3. Don't reprimand them if they are late for an appointment or phone call.

4. Be encouraging about what they can do to help their family member.

5. Acknowledge their "cheerleader" status with the patient.

"Everything can be taken from a man but one thing: the last of human freedoms—to choose one's attitude in any given set of circumstances, to choose one's own way."
—Viktor Emil Frankl, MD, PhD

Difficult Patients With Bad Attitudes

Your Brain Color personality might clash with a patient's Brain Colors when he or she exhibits a bad attitude and/or are difficult to care for. The following will offer insight into patients' attitudes and behaviors:

- **Yellow Brain** patients' bad attitude may be caused by a sense of worry and not being in control of their health care. They can be difficult to care for because of their unwillingness to change their behavior. You can help these patients by involving them in the development of their health care plan. Feeling in control will improve the patients' attitude and make them feel safer and more secure that they are being cared for in "the right way."

- **Blue Brain** patients' bad attitude may be caused by their uncomfortable feeling of not being listened to. They can be difficult to care for because they require a lot of time to talk about their emotions concerning their health. You can help these patients improve their attitude by scheduling a reasonable amount of time to listen to their concerns and talking about why they are distressed about their health, which will make them feel that you genuinely care about them.

- **Green Brain** patients' bad attitude may be caused by a lack of information about their care. They can be difficult to care for because they think the people who are caring for them are incompetent. You can help these patients by offering them specific background information about the health care professionals who are involved in their care. Offering them the appropriate research data about their health issues will improve their attitude. This knowledge will give them the ability able to speak intelligently about their health concerns.

- **Orange Brain** patients' bad attitude may be caused by the restrictions their poor health has caused. They can be difficult to care for because they do not like being told what to do and how to do it. You can help these patients improve their attitude by developing a health care plan that will give them immediate results, which will instantly reward them, such as when they received gold stars on a spelling chart when they were in school.

Generational Misunderstandings

To avoid the generational misunderstandings between you, your patients, and their family members, it will be helpful to recognize and understand what each generation values.

Silent Generation or War Babies, who were born between 1925 and 1945, value hard work, respect for authority, commitment, responsibility, and deferential patient care.

Baby Boomers, who were born between 1946 and 1962, value loyalty, traditions, respect for ones' reputation, security, and considerate patient care.

Generation X, who were born between 1963 and 1980, value caution, inquiry, taking care of themselves, and receiving good service for their money and efficient patient care.

Generation Y, who were born between 1981 and 2000, value confidence, optimism, communication, involvement, responsiveness, and pragmatic patient care.

Understanding these generational differences and the Brain Color approach will help you to avoid misunderstandings and to build a cooperative relationship with your patients and their family members. Remember the following four generational tips:

1. Recognize and be flexible about what each generation values, even if what they value is different from what you regard as valuable.

2. Do not judge a generation by their appearance, get to know who they are and discover their Brain Color personality.

3. Keep an open mind about diversity, generational attitudes, and Brain Color behaviors.

4. Adapt and modify your Brain Color approach to accommodate and communicate with different generation patients and their family members.

Family Members' Feelings

Adult and pediatric patients' family members play a significant role in your patients' health care. Patients' family members may complain because they feel dismissed if they have to chase a health care professional down the hall to get an update about their loved one, are told they do not need to know, do not have their questions answered, and/or are treated as if they are invisible. Keep in mind that family members of your adult and pediatric patients may find it difficult to be:

- Courageous when they are frightened.
- Strong when they are exhausted.
- Prepared when they are overwhelmed.
- Composed when they are angry.
- Supportive when they are disappointed.
- Esteemed when they are frustrated.
- Communicative when they want to cry.
- Patient when they are confused.
- Self-caring when feeling that there are not enough hours in the day to manage their loved one's care, not to mention taking care of themselves.

Primary Caregiver's Tips

by Laura R. Palgon, MEd

When my mother was ill, there were many times when she was rushed to the emergency room. As her primary caregiver and as a new mother myself, I was in a position where my Yellow/Blue Brain needed to be ready for anything at a moment's notice.

There were two things I did to prepare for our frequent emergencies. These things helped to alleviate stress for me as the caregiver, allowing me to focus my attention on my mother and her needs.

First, I created a comprehensive, succinct, and easy to read emergency medical history document for my mother, including the names and telephone numbers of all of her doctors, a current list of her medications and dosages, and a list of all of her allergies, surgeries and conditions. I also included insurance information and emergency contact names and telephone numbers. I made many copies of this document and put it in envelopes marked EMERGENCY INFORMATION in bold red letters. Because my mother lived alone, I worried that something might happen when I was not available to help her. I put copies of that emergency medical history document everywhere! My mother carried one in her purse and in her car. There was one posted on the refrigerator in her home. Both my husband and I each kept one in our cars. There were many times this document came in handy.

Arriving at the emergency room is hectic and scary. The hospital needs insurance and medical information before they can help you. But all you want is help for your loved one! How frustrating it can be to remember all that complicated information when you are so concerned with your loved one's health. Upon arriving to the emergency room, I would hand this document to the intake nurse, who was happy to have everything so clearly presented. This made the intake process so much easier and faster! My mother was seen and cared for just a few minutes sooner, and that can make a big difference. For me, as the caregiver, having this document helped to calm a stressful situation.

The second thing I did to prepare for the random, yet frequent, emergencies was put together a bag just for emergencies. I called it my "Go Bag." It was filled with items for my baby if we had to suddenly leave the house to help my mother or take her to the emergency room. The "Go Bag" included diapers, toys, and snacks for the baby and a book for me. Most importantly, it included the emergency medical history document.

It is not easy to care for a family member who needs frequent help, so anything you can do to calm a chaotic situation is worth doing! Having a plan, being prepared, and providing medical staff with current and accurate information can make all the difference for the person you love.

Patient Advocates

It will make your job easier, more rewarding, and successful when patients feel that their health care professional treats them with respect and fairness, communicates clearly, and offers them beneficial knowledge to make them feel informed, comfortable, and more engaged and committed to their own health care plan. Patients also feel more secure when they have a "Patient Advocate" or "Think Partner," who also feels cared about and secure to make critical health care decisions with and for the patient.

- When you are taking care of your patients, you are often also taking care of their concerned partners, children, family members, friends, and/or advocates. You might be offering them information about their loved one and comfort, understanding, and/or awareness about their loved one's health that they did not know.

- Your patient might also need another type of patient advocate, who could be a case manager, social worker, nurse, trained health care professional, or a former doctor, who can help a patient with health care plans or government-provided services, transition to assistant living facilities or nursing homes, and provide transportation, bill tracking, and payment assistance.

- You or your staff may have to communicate or collaborate with government consumer patient advocacy agencies that offer services to your patients. These agencies are responsible for developing policies and legislation to improve systems or processes for patients, such as not-for-profit health care or specific disease associations or societies.

Whether you are working with an individual and/or an agency or association staff member, understanding their Brain Color perspective regarding how to approach them and develop a beneficial relationship with them is critical to your patients' health care and well-being.

Remember to add a smile to your approach and see what happens!

A Smile For Your Patients

Keep your smiled pinned on!
It may give another cheer;
It may soothe another's fear;
It may help another fight,
If your smile's tight!
—Anonymous

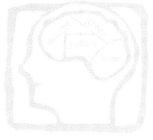

YOUR RELATIONSHIP
WITH COWORKERS

Who Done It?

Once upon a time, there were four people.
Their names were Everybody, Somebody, Nobody and Anybody.
Whenever there was an important job to be done,
Everybody was sure that Somebody would do it.
Anybody could have done it, but Nobody did it.
When Nobody did it, Everybody got angry because it was
Everybody's job.
Everybody thought that Somebody would do it,
But Nobody realized that Nobody would do it.
So consequently Everybody blamed Somebody when Nobody did
what Anybody could have done in the first place.
—Anonymous

In this chapter, you will examine coworkers' Brain Color attributes to build collaborative relationships and create harmony between the Brain Colors to increase productive teamwork, offer excellent care to your patients, and complete your tasks compassionately and efficiently.

From *What Color Is Your Brain?® When Caring for Patients:*
An Easy Approach for Understanding Your
Personality Type and Your Patient's Perspective.
Published by SLACK Incorporated.

YELLOW BRAIN COWORKER'S ATTRIBUTES

MY WORK ATTITUDE: Be practical

I SEE MYSELF AS: Punctual

WITH MY TEAM: I am a detailed leader

I MAKE DECISIONS: In a timely manner

MY PRIORITY IS: Reliability

WHEN FRUSTRATED: I worry

MY COLLABORATIVE POINT OF VIEW: Respectfulness

I NEED: A sense of orderliness

I ACCOMPLISH GOALS BY: Being prepared

ACKNOWLEDGE MY: Accountability

 GREEN BRAIN COWORKER'S ATTRIBUTES

MY WORK ATTITUDE: Be methodical

I SEE MYSELF AS: Intelligent

WITH MY TEAM: I am a composed problem solver

I MAKE DECISIONS: By researching the facts

MY PRIORITY IS: Efficiency

WHEN FRUSTRATED: I withdraw

MY COLLABORATIVE POINT OF VIEW: Fairness

I NEED: Privacy to process my thoughts

I ACCOMPLISH GOALS BY: Developing systems

ACKNOWLEDGE MY: Competency

BLUE BRAIN COWORKER'S ATTRIBUTES

MY WORK ATTITUDE: Be adaptable

I SEE MYSELF AS: Creative

WITH MY TEAM: I am a helpful nurturer

I MAKE DECISIONS: After talking with others

MY PRIORITY IS: Cooperation

WHEN FRUSTRATED: I say I am "fine" but I'm not

MY COLLABORATIVE POINT OF VIEW: Teamwork

I NEED: To share my ideas

I ACCOMPLISH GOALS BY: Asking others to help

ACKNOWLEDGE MY: Compassion

 ORANGE BRAIN COWORKER'S ATTRIBUTES

MY WORK ATTITUDE: Be a troubleshooter

I SEE MYSELF AS: Dynamic

WITH MY TEAM: I am a fun team player

I MAKE DECISIONS: In the moment

MY PRIORITY IS: Results

WHEN FRUSTRATED: I say, "I am out of here!"

MY COLLABORATIVE POINT OF VIEW: Energetic

I NEED: Freedom for self-expression

I ACCOMPLISH GOALS BY: Taking risks

ACKNOWLEDGE MY: Positive outlook

The Little Yellow Canary

During a staff development program, it was evident that the Orange Brainers agitated the Yellow Brainers. One of the Yellow Brain team members said, "We're misunderstood and unappreciated. The Orange Brainers do *not* value timeliness, they mock our organizational requirements, and they are clueless about our needs."

An Orange Brainer said, "We're concerned with getting the results we need, not the procedures that are on someone else's schedule."

After lunch, a Yellow Brainer, who had been an English teacher in a previous career, read the following poem to the workshop participants:

We Yellow people are feeling very Blue,
Because of all the nasty things that were said about us.
We're Green with envy over all the positive attributes the
rest of you seem to have.
Now, Orange, are you ashamed of yourselves for putting us down?

Signed,
Joan Fessler, Sweet, Nurturing, Intelligent, Fun-loving Little Canary

The Orange Brainers got the point and reciprocated. At the close of the program, an Orange Brainer recited his poem:

The Orange Brainers need to have fun,
But without the Yellow Brainers nothing would get done!

The information in this chapter will examine your coworkers' Brain Color attributes and help you to understand how to connect with your coworkers to build relationships, understand their attributes, harmoniously collaborate with them, and understand their frustrations according to their Brain Colors.

Work in Perfect Harmony

A staff team building program at Community Crisis Center in Elgin, Illinois, which is one of the oldest domestic violence shelters in the state of Illinois, was a perfect example of perfect harmony. The meeting room reverberated with laughter when the staff members completed their Brain Color Quizzes. The noise level quickly elevated while they stuck their Yellow, Blue, Green, and Orange dots on their name tags. Those moments of discovery are the prelude to a lively chorus of exclamations and harmonious banter, such as:

"Oh, Michelle and I are exactly the same colors, no wonder we work so well together!"

"Now I know why I have such a hard time getting along with and working with John; he's so Green and I'm so Blue!"

"I understand why my Orange needs Maureen's Yellow to get the job done!"

"It's incredible, that's why our team works in perfect harmony!"

The Crisis Center staff members speak fluent Brain Color and have incorporated the concept into their professional lives. I love the frequent Brain Color messages from Maureen Manning-Rosenfeld, who is the Yellow/Blue Brain Director of Client Services at the Crisis Center.

One day, I received the following email message from Maureen:

> Your ears must have been ringing yesterday! I am actually getting really good at predicting someone's Brain Color before they announce it! We had a funny moment when one of the professionals, a male social worker who's been in the field for 30+ years, told the interns, "Don't worry, you'll change." He tested as follows: Orange-Green-Yellow-Blue!!!
>
> I also used the information to explain that the different Brain Colors approach crisis intervention differently. There is no wrong way, just different approaches. AND the beauty of the team here is that different counselors click with different clients—for instance, on our 8 to 4 shift, we have a Green Supervisor, one Yellow Case Manager, and one Blue Case Manager. One of the new staff members

commented that thinking back to my lecture on professional ethics from the day before, she could see how the Yellow staff help the Blues from crossing over their boundaries from professional to personal relationships. It clicked! As ever, thanks for your body of work, which has helped improve the services that we provide here.

I'm Frustrated!

It's easier to promote harmony and increase productivity when your coworkers' frustrations are recognized and acknowledged and when their perspective is valued.

The Coworkers' Brain Color Frustrations chart on page 77 will help you recognize your coworkers' frustrations that lead to negative behavior. The Brain Color Teamwork Behavior Charts on pages 78 and 79 will help you understand how to manage and encourage cooperative behavior to develop positive and compatible relationships in your workplace.

Brain Color Frustrations

Yellow Brain Frustrations	Blue Brain Frustrations	Green Brain Frustrations	Orange Brain Frustrations
Not being in control	Apathy	Intrusions	Someone else's schedule
Disorder	Inconsideration	Redundancy	Never enough time
Lack of preparation	Ineffective communication	Not seeing the big picture	No action or results
Irresponsibility	Dishonesty	Incomplete data	Whining
Tardiness	Insensitivity	No forethought	Pessimism
Distractions	Conflict	Technical systems down	Waiting
Poor or no instructions	Lack of cooperation	Absence of independent thinking	Void of energy

From *What Color Is Your Brain?® When Caring for Patients: An Easy Approach for Understanding Your Personality Type and Your Patient's Perspective.* Published by SLACK Incorporated. Copyright Sheila N. Glazov. http://www.sheilaglazov.com

YELLOW BRAIN TEAMWORK BEHAVIOR

Offers a "Well done" pat on the back

Says, "Nice job!"

Offers awards

Follows the rules to outcome

Is respectful toward others

Minimizes arguments

Decreases confrontations

Affirms with acknowledgments

Asks for and uses input

 GREEN BRAIN TEAMWORK BEHAVIOR

Thinks of unique solutions

Offers financial acknowledgments

Methodically accomplishes tasks

Examines alternatives

Thrives on new challenges

Considers consequences

Does not accept excuses from others

Is pragmatic

Acknowledges innovative ideas

BLUE BRAIN TEAMWORK BEHAVIOR

Offers encouragement

Inspires others

Shares creative ideas

Is mutually considerate

Acknowledges gratefulness

Does not like gossip

Is truthful

Thanks others frequently

Gives hugs when appropriate

 ORANGE BRAIN TEAMWORK BEHAVIOR

Gets results quickly

Has fun on the job

Gives validation freely

Highly competitive

Respects nonconformity

Does not like "wet blankets"

Is not a "nay sayer"

Defends coworkers

Supports coworkers' opinions

Coworkers' Brain Color Frustrations

You will no longer have to think of your coworkers as prima donnas whose negative behavior frustrates you. The following list will help you to deal with that behavior and show your coworkers compassion and concern.

Yellow Brainers

- Speak frankly about what they see.
- Attempt to understand coworkers' expectations.
- Are patient.
- Are respectful.

Blue Brainers

- Are empathetic with coworkers.
- Model appropriate behavior.
- Ask coworkers how they can help them.
- Listen to the coworker's side of the story

Green Brainers

- Ignore coworkers' behavior and not meddle.
- Let coworkers know they value their explanation.
- Try not to be too critical.
- Respect coworkers' privacy if they do not want to talk.

Orange Brainers

- Give coworkers their space.
- Ask coworkers to explain why they are frustrated.
- Walk away from the situation.
- Consider what might be going on in a coworker's personal life.

Newbie and Veteran

Teaching and training a new health care employee (Newbie) how to work with a long-time veteran (Vet) team member often can be challenging. Each Newbie and Vet will have a different Brain Color perspective about how to handle this sensitive transition.

 YELLOW BRAIN VETERAN PERSPECTIVE

- Orient Newbies about procedures and become their mentor.
- Include Newbies in decision making and problem solving.

 BLUE BRAIN VETERAN PERSPECTIVE

- Help Newbies feel like they are part of the team.
- Make sure that the Newbies feel secure about their new knowledge and feel comfortable to ask questions of the Vets at another time.

 GREEN BRAIN VETERAN PERSPECTIVE

- Orient Newbies about strategies to become familiar with new information.
- Vets instruct Newbies about technology.

 ORANGE BRAIN VETERAN PERSPECTIVE

- Help Newbies feel like they can approach Vets with any questions.
- Create a buddy system for Newbies to help one another.

Accountable Teamwork

One complaint I often hear when clients are discussing issues within their organization is: "We want to develop more teamwork and accountability, so we can do things better." To develop the teamwork they desire, team members need to know how to encourage accountability with one another by understanding what each Brain Color needs to be accountable to his or her other team members.

YELLOW BRAINERS NEED

- Detailed lists of policies
- Assignment of tasks, goals, and timelines
- To promote communication with follow-up actions
- To provide appropriate resources to complete tasks on time

BLUE BRAINERS NEED

- Positive feedback
- Group discussions
- Others to listen to them
- To allow others to do things in their own **creative** manner

GREEN BRAINERS NEED

- Resources to keep accurate research
- Time to think about problems and solutions
- A methodology when offering their own innovative solutions to a problem
- To work by themselves or one-to-one with others

ORANGE BRAINERS NEED

- To get to the point quickly
- Others to hear their opinion, even if it sounds silly
- To be asked, "What needs to be done right away?"
- No time wasted talking when they could be doing

It's a Puzzlement

During a pre-workshop meeting, my client confided in me, saying, "One of my most competent managers totally mystifies me. I am at a loss for words to describe his baffling behavior. He's driving me crazy! His staff is so frustrated and bewildered that every day one of them wants to quit. I hired him because he was referred to me with glowing professional references, but I didn't realize that his interpersonal skills were so inadequate."

After a deep breath, she continued, "How was I to know that he would behave like a raving tyrant when things just didn't go his way or one of his staff members would dare to give him a suggestion?"

"Sounds like you have a puzzle that is missing a few significant pieces," I suggested.

"Only a few?" she chuckled. "To look at him or see him in action with a client you would not believe we were talking about the same person. But how do I find the missing pieces to the puzzle?"

"It's simple," I assured her. "The solution is in understanding the manager's Brain Color and the staff members' perspective."

When problems arise, think of your coworkers as if they were a multipiece puzzle that needs to be solved.

The Puzzlement Solution

If you are unable to solve the problem that perplexes you, the solution becomes as complicated as a 1,000-piece picture puzzle. However, if you utilize the Brain Color Coworkers' Attributes charts on pages 72-73, the puzzle becomes easy to solve.

To be collaborative, productive, and successful in your health care workplace, spend time discovering the puzzle pieces of your Brain Color perspective and your coworkers' point of view. If you understand how to put the colorful pieces together and fit them into the appropriate places, you will decrease frustration, increase cooperation, and solve puzzlements in your workplace. You will also develop mutually caring relationships with your coworkers.

My "Coworker Family" Saved My Life!

by Tom Garcia, RRT, RCP

Tom, Respiratory Care Practitioner (RCP): "As an RCP, I had worked at a large city hospital for more than half of my life and was familiar with the diverse population of the staff. However, being a health care worker doesn't always make a person vigilant about their own well-being. I had been having abdominal pain for some time, and it seemed to be getting worse. Like so many men, I ignored the pain, made excuses, and was in denial. I never had a serious health problem in my life. I had never been hospitalized. I didn't even have a primary physician."

Mimi, RCP Supervisor: However, procrastination, an old friend, won out. Until one day, after giving a nebulizer treatment in a patient's room, I felt a sudden sharp pain in my lower left abdomen. By the time I arrived at my supervisor's office, the pain was intense. I told my supervisor that I was having some abdominal pain and wanted to go home and rest. Fortunately, the supervisor had better judgment. She looked at me calmly and firmly, said, *"You are not going anywhere, except to the ED [emergency department]."*

Norman, ED Head Nurse: Norman, the ED nurse, immediately led me to the trauma room, where I had spent the majority of my time with the trauma team intubating and initiating mechanical ventilation on every type of trauma patient. After I described the pain, James' Orange resourceful brain wasted no time getting an IV [intravenous therapy] started and summoning the trauma team. The gravity of the situation began to sink in.

Dr. Singhal, Trauma Chief: When the trauma chief arrived, his Green/Orange Brain approach immediately gathered information and ordered tests, including a CT [computerized tomography] scan. His Blue Brain reassured me that he would be back after the CT results were available. After the CT scan, the trauma chief returned to my trauma room and said, *"Well it looks like you bought yourself some surgery."*

Lizbeth, Trauma Nurse: The following day, Lizbeth, a trauma nurse and a former nurse practitioner in the respiratory care department, came to my room to reassure me that she would coordinate my surgery and postoperative care.

Dr. Sanchez, Radiologist: In the Interventional Radiology Department, the radiologist was the best example of someone who was firing on all his Brain Colors. He began explaining the procedure to me in a Green Brain comprehensive manner without being condescending or aloof. When he saw the apprehension on my face, he told me, *"Everything will be fine. We're going to take care of you, don't worry! You're part of this family."*

Chief Resident, who shall remain nameless: That night I met the unforgettable chief resident on call. He was a Green Brainer to the core. All day, my pain increased. After a quick examination, another CT was ordered, and pain medication would be administered throughout the night. However, the radiology department was extremely busy; there was a miscommunication, delays, and more pain. I requested pain medication, but the chief resident allowed only a maintenance dose. I demanded to see him! The resident dramatically stood in the doorway as I explained that the trauma service had approved more pain medication if I needed it. My Blue Intuitive Brain realized that the resident was suspicious of my motives to obtain more pain medication. He asserted his authority, refused to give me any stronger medications, and left me suffering in excruciating pain.

Jorge, Radiology Technician: I was becoming depressed until the radiology technician arrived. He could not believe that I was the last patient. Neither of us understood why I had waited so long to be taken for the scan.

Dr. Singhal and Lizbeth: The next few days were filled with more tests, x-rays, and an MRI [magnetic resonance imaging], but there was no improvement, and new pain developed due to an infection. Dr. Singhal told me about his plan for a high-risk surgical procedure. I asked Lizbeth to stay when Dr. Singhal left the room. I asked her how serious my condition was. Her Yellow/Green Brain objectively replied, *"It's serious, but not that serious."*

Nursing Staff, Trauma Team, and Transporter: The next few days were filled with preparation for the surgery. I noticed how Green Brain and Yellow Brain the nursing staff and trauma team were. I was lucky! All my coworkers were giving me exceptional care, which made being a patient a lot less frightening. On the morning of the surgery, Frank, the transporter, came to take me to the OR [operating room]. His personality was bursting with Orange optimism as he told me, "Tom, I have no doubt whatsoever that everything will be fine!"

Dr. Jeong, Anesthesiologist: When Frank and I arrived at the pre-operative suite, the anesthesiologist, Dr. Jeong, was there with his soothing Blue Brain manner and voice, which was comforting as I drifted into an anesthetic abyss.

Maria, Recovery Room Nurse: In what seemed like a very short time, I was awakened by Maria's voice telling *me*, "Take deep breaths." Words I had said to hundreds of patients in the RR [recovery room]. Now, I was on the other side of the rail. As soon as I could form the words, I ask Maria what most patients ask immediately after their surgery, *"How did it go?"*

My surgery was successful! Not only did I appreciate the extraordinary care I received, I appreciated the tender and terrorizing lessons I learned as a patient. Now I understood and knew how patients feel when they are cared for compassionately, when they suffer pain, intimidation, and fear. Most of all, I am grateful that my Coworker Family saved my life!

Now that you have learned to recognize and *see* your coworkers' Brain Color attributes, cooperative behavior, frustrations, and components for successful teamwork, it will be easier for you to effectively connect with them and build harmonious relationships.

It is also essential to remember Anaïs Nin's cautionary quote:

> *"We don't see things as they are. We see them as we are."*

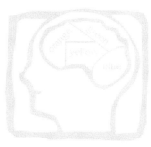

YOUR RELATIONSHIP WITH MANAGEMENT (LEADERS, MANAGERS, AND ADMINISTRATORS) AND AGENCIES

Achieving Goals Successfully

by Michael Epstein, MD

Today's academic medical centers are large, complex, multifaceted organizations in which various stakeholders share some, but not all, of their goals and objectives. Managing the trade-offs between the aspirations and needs of these various stakeholders (physicians, nurses, nonprofessional staff, patients and their families, regulators, payors, and the Board of Trustees) while ensuring the highest quality of care, maximum access, and enough of a "profit margin" to ensure that the financial well-being of the institution falls to the executive team leading the medical center and, in terms of day-to-day operations, to the chief operating officer.

In the chief operating officer role for 5 years at the Beth Israel Deaconess Medical Center, one of Harvard Medical School's major teaching hospitals, I had the intellectually stimulating, but often frustratingly difficult, opportunity to try to meld those conflicting goals, achieving unity of purpose and action at this 600+ bed, $1.25 billion per year operation.

One example of a situation where we were able to achieve agreement among these different stakeholders, each with their own "personality," goals, and objectives, was the opening of a satellite outpatient specialty center in a Boston suburb. The hospital's goal was to deliver high quality care in a setting convenient for patients, who could avoid the trip, traffic, and parking in downtown Boston and still access our skilled physicians and nurses. Although embracing the goal, our physician groups were hesitant to make the commitment to staff the new center. Primarily Green in their brain orientation, they tended to be conservative and cautious in undertaking new investments and creative projects. The nurses also were hesitant. Although primarily Blue in their compassionate and communicative styles, they were also uncertain of the practice standards and logistics in a new and distant location. It fell to me, Yellow in my organized, punctual, and responsible nature, to get all the parties to the table and reach agreement.

The center opened and has been a major success—good for patients, good for the physicians who have grown their practices, and good for the hospital and its employees, including the nurses, as we have gained a market share and increased revenues. This successful model has been replicated in additional suburban centers as a positive strategy in a complex and challenging environment.

Successful Relationships

The Brain Color approach helps individuals successfully connect with and build relationships with the leaders, managers, and administrators in their medical center or office and the health care agency representatives with whom they work every day. To achieve and maintain successful relationships, it is essential to understand and respect each Brain Color attributes and perspective and how each Brain Color sees the other Brain Colors' attributes and abilities.

"I have learned that success is to be measured not so much by the position that one has reached in life as by the obstacles which he has overcome while trying to succeed."
—Booker T. Washington

The Rapidly Changing Workplace

In the today's workplace, it seems that individuals are metaphorically rollerblading at a high speed and being regulated by an increasing number of agencies. Currently, leaders, managers, and administrators need to adapt to their rapidly changing workplace, work more effectively with their team members, and build cooperative relationships with agency representatives. Those individuals can be more successful if they recognize and understand their Brain Color personality type and others' traits and talents and know how to deal with change, make decisions effectively, and interact with other individuals collaboratively. Health care leaders, managers, administrators, and agency representatives will be more successful, work more collaboratively, and achieve their goals faster when they recognize and utilize their Brain Color knowledge when working with other individuals in their health care facility.

 Yellow Brain Leaders, Managers, Administrators, and Agency Representatives

- **Yellow Brainers** are disciplined, sensible, and contribute stability and structure to an organization.
- They are goal-oriented with their team members.
- They have a realistic approach with agency representatives.
- They require a plan to feel comfortable about changes and need to know they are in control of the circumstances.
- To adapt to change and make decisions, they must work in an organized environment where tasks are completed on time, and they must know what is expected of themselves and others.
- If they are not able to easily adapt to the changes, they become anxious, judgmental, and/or inflexible.

Blue Brain Leaders, Managers, Administrators, and Agency Representatives

- **Blue Brainers** are nurturing, inspiring, and contribute friendliness and interaction to an organization.
- They are encouraging with their team members.
- They are considerate of agency representatives.
- They need to intuitively feel comfortable about change and making decisions after they have listened and communicated with each team member.
- To adapt to change and make decisions, they must work in a collaborative environment that promotes harmony, imagination, and flexibility among all the participants.
- If they are not able to easily adapt to the changes, they become depressed, overly sensitive, and/or unrealistic.

 Green Brain Leaders, Managers, Administrators, and Agency Representatives

- **Green Brainers** are mentally focused visionaries who contribute strategy and innovation to an organization.
- They prefer to work independently, rather than with their team members.
- They are not talkative and give only the facts to agency representatives.
- They need to gather data to feel comfortable about change and make decisions after they analyze all pertinent information.
- To adapt to change and make decisions, they need to work independently in a tranquil environment, which promotes efficiency, competence, research, and the latest technology.
- If they are not able to easily adapt to the changes, they become intolerant, noncommunicative and/or intimidating.

Orange Brain Leaders, Managers, Administrators, and Agency Representatives

- **Orange Brainers** are results-oriented, skillful negotiators who contribute excitement and adaptability to the organization.
- They encourage competition among their team members.
- They can be helpful troubleshooters with agency representatives.
- They are change agents and feel comfortable creating change and making decisions spontaneously and optimistically.
- To adapt to change and make decisions, they must work at their own pace without a lot of structure in a virtual environment, promoting open-mindedness, competition, and freedom to be self-reliant.
- If they are not able to easily adapt to the changes, they become impulsive, rude, and/or emotionally explosive.

Often, an obstacle to success is another individual's perspective of a goal that must be achieved. The following *Leadership and Management Attributes* and *Perspectives of Leaders, Manager, Administrators, and Agency Representatives* charts demonstrate each Brain Color's perspective and how each Brain Color see the other Colors' point of view.

YELLOW BRAIN LEADERSHIP AND MANAGEMENT ATTRIBUTES

I AM: Practical

I VALUE: Dedication

I AM RESPONSIBLE FOR: Coaching team members

I STEP UP TO RESPONSIBILITY: With initiative

I WORK EFFECTIVELY BY: Being organized

I DELEGATE TASKS BY: Giving assignments

I GET THE JOB DONE BY: Being prepared and prompt

WORKING WITH AGENCIES: I keep perfect records

I ACHIEVE MY GOALS BY: Following an exact plan

GREEN BRAIN LEADERSHIP AND MANAGEMENT ATTRIBUTES

I AM: Methodical

I VALUE: Efficient processes

I AM RESPONSIBLE FOR: Giving parameters to my team

I STEP UP TO RESPONSIBILITY: With competency

I WORK EFFECTIVELY BY: Being objective

I DELEGATE TASKS BY: Being fair minded

I GET THE JOB DONE BY: Using evidence-based facts

WORKING WITH AGENCIES: I offer my expertise

I ACHIEVE MY GOALS BY: Scrutinizing the resources

BLUE BRAIN LEADERSHIP AND MANAGEMENT ATTRIBUTES

I AM: Adaptable

I VALUE: "Out-of-the-box" thinking

I AM RESPONSIBLE FOR: Encouraging team members

I STEP UP TO RESPONSIBILITY: With enthusiasm

I WORK EFFECTIVELY BY: Expressing my ideas

I DELEGATE TASKS BY: Asking others to help

I GET THE JOB DONE BY: Being a sincere listener

WORKING WITH AGENCIES: I create trustworthiness

I ACHIEVE MY GOALS BY: Promoting cooperation

ORANGE BRAIN LEADERSHIP AND MANAGEMENT ATTRIBUTES

I AM: Confident

I VALUE: Receptiveness to new ideas

I AM RESPONSIBLE FOR: Being a team resource

I STEP UP TO RESPONSIBILITY: With momentum

I WORK EFFECTIVELY BY: Focusing on results

I DELEGATE TASKS BY: My team taking ownership

I GET THE JOB DONE BY: Creating competition

WORKING WITH AGENCIES: I am congenial

I ACHIEVE MY GOALS BY: Energizing my team

From *What Color Is Your Brain?® When Caring for Patients: An Easy Approach for Understanding Your Personality Type and Your Patient's Perspective.* Published by SLACK Incorporated. Copyright Sheila N. Glazov. http://www.sheilaglazov.com

Yellow Brainers' Perspective of Leaders, Managers, Administrators, and Agency Representatives			
Yellow Brainers See Yellow Brainers as:	Yellow Brainers See Blue Brainers as:	Yellow Brainers See Green Brainers as:	Yellow Brainers See Orange Brainers as:
Dependable	Warm	Brainy	Risk takers
Effective	Genuine	Thorough	Self-starters
Practical	Sincere	Focused	Clever
Resistant to change	Disorganized	Insensitive	Immature
Dedicated	Chatty	Secretive	Uncooperative
Serious	Ambiguous	Condescending	Erratic

From *What Color Is Your Brain?® When Caring for Patients: An Easy Approach for Understanding Your Personality Type and Your Patient's Perspective.* Published by SLACK Incorporated. Copyright Sheila N. Glazov. http://www.sheilaglazov.com

Blue Brainers' Perspective of Leaders, Managers, Administrators, and Agency Representatives			
Blue Brainers See Blue Brainers as:	**Blue Brainers See Yellow Brainers as:**	**Blue Brainers See Green Brainers as:**	**Blue Brainers See Orange Brainers as:**
Compassionate	Determined	Methodical	Spontaneous
Authentic	Perfectionists	Independent	Resourceful
Family focused	List makers	Logical	Change agents
Creative	Bossy	Uncommunicative	Procrastinators
Good listeners	Doing it themselves	Unreasonable	Innovative
Accommodating	Demanding	Emotionally cold	Inconsiderate

From *What Color Is Your Brain? When Caring for Patients: An Easy Approach for Understanding Your Personality Type and Your Patient's Perspective.* Published by SLACK Incorporated. Copyright Sheila N. Glazov. http://www.sheilaglazov.com

Green Brainers' Perspective of Leaders, Managers, Administrators, and Agency Representatives			
Green Brainers See Green Brainers as:	**Green Brainers See Yellow Brainers as:**	**Green Brainers See Blue Brainers as:**	**Green Brainers See Orange Brainers as:**
Intelligent	Conventional	Forgiving	Funny
Objective	Reliable	Harmonious	Energetic
Rational	Disciplinarians	Inspirational	Ingenious
Bottom line counts	Worriers	Scattered	Unpredictable
To the point	Finicky	Contradictory	Disruptive
Judicious	Practical	Arbitrary	Show offs

From *What Color Is Your Brain?® When Caring for Patients: An Easy Approach for Understanding Your Personality Type and Your Patient's Perspective*. Published by SLACK Incorporated. Copyright Sheila N. Glazov. http://www.sheilaglazov.com

Orange Brainers' Perspective of Leaders, Managers, Administrators, and Agency Representatives			
Orange Brainers See Orange Brainers as:	Orange Brainers See Yellow Brainers as:	Orange Brainers See Blue Brainers as:	Orange Brainers See Green Brainers as:
Entertaining	Structured	Nurturing	Smart
Exciting	Prompt	Trusting	Technical
Persuasive	Boring	Imaginative	Instructive
Hands on	Rigid	Meddlesome	Sticklers
Getting results quickly	Interfering	Passive	Standoffish
Amicable	Bureaucratic	Conflicted	Aloof

Community Care

by Clint C. Parram, MPH

I am a Green Brain Problem Solver, and the association I work for requires annual safety program assessments for the hospitals who are clients of our group. During one of these visits, my contact, the Yellow Brain Human Resources Director, and I were touring the hospital when I became aware of a slightly acidic odor.

The human resources director informed me that the construction the hospital was undergoing at times produced the odor. Discussions with the construction foreman had not gone well. He had indicated that the renovation required the application of certain chemicals and that the odor was unavoidable.

The issue was significant enough that we decided the CEO [chief executive officer] of the hospital should be advised of the situation. The Blue Brain CEO, a very accessible individual and an open communicator, immediately let us interrupt his day. After hearing our concerns for employee and patient safety, the CEO took immediate action. Although the actions disrupted the renovation project and added extra costs, the chemical exposure was eliminated, and the caring and healing environment was maintained.

This particular hospital is classified as small and rural and is a major employer in the city. Therefore, the ratio of employees having loved ones being treated here is much higher than in a mid- to large-size suburban or city hospital. The hospital really is a "community" hospital!

From my Green Brain Agency Perspective, I have observed the following:

- Community hospital staff members, leaders, managers, and administrators appear to be more accepting of construction inconveniences than their counterparts in a large "city" hospital might be.

- The relationship of local construction company workers, who may be family members, friends, and/or neighbors of the community hospital staff, definitely influences what or if negative comments are made about the work being done in the hospital.

Rounding and Relationships

You do not have to work in a hospital to implement "Rounding" in your health care facility. The term *Rounding* refers to:

- Building clear communication within a health care organization.
- Engaging team members to offer their ideas and improvements.
- Identifying and acknowledging the events and individuals that positively impact the health care organization and environment.
- An ongoing focus of changing and/or improving staff members' skills, attitudes, and safety, as well as patients' comfort, care, and safety.

To implement Rounding, health care management (leaders and managers) in a hospital or health care facility need to be visible (at different times of the day). While rounding, these leaders and managers need to be able to approach and engage team members and patients to learn meaningful, relevant, and significant information, thus building trust by listening and responding to their concerns. The following are examples of Brain Color Rounding:

Yellow Brainers' Management Rounding: Making sure everything is being done according to the rules.

Blue Brainers' Management Rounding: Listening to staff members and patients encourages them and lets them know you care.

Green Brainers' Management Rounding: Gathering all the facts and checking out the latest technology.

Orange Brainers' Management Rounding: Interacting with patients and staff members.

Successful **"Brainbow" Rounding** is a combination of leaders' and managers' Brain Colors' Rounding behaviors.

Four Keys to Effective Administrative Rounding

The following are excerpts from the article *4 Keys to Effective Administrative Rounding* written by J. Stephen Lindsey, FACHE, and Brett Corkran. The four keys are also included in the book *Take Charge of Your Healthcare Management Career: 50 Lessons That Drive Success* by J. Stephen Lindsey and Kenneth R. White. The lessons demonstrate the effectiveness of Rounding.

Alexander the Great was famous for riding his horse among his ranks of soldiers before combat, calling out individuals by name and exalting their bravery in prior battles. He connected with individuals and inspired his army as a whole when he rode into battle with them. Hospital administrators can learn much from this leadership style. Though it is advisable to leave the horse at home, administrative Rounding has become a key to successful management over the years. In the late 1970s, Tom Peters coined the term *"management by walking around."* The Japanese know it as taking the "Gemba Walk," and Quint Studer is famous for his "Rounding for Outcomes." No matter what it is called though, the same core principles of hospital rounding remain steadfast.

1. Commitment

"Unless commitment is made, there are only promises and hopes ... but no plans." —Peter Drucker, management consultant and author

Get out of your office! ... Any opportunity to be more visible within your organization should be utilized .... It provides a chance to develop rapport with co-workers and glean insight from casual conversation.... Attempting to bridge the divide between administration and clinicians is not an easy task, but it is indispensable to quality leadership. Employees want leaders who share the same goals and are willing to struggle alongside them to achieve success. Committing to rounding as a daily necessity is a crucial first step in better connecting with your organization.

2. Observation

"You can observe a lot just by watching." —Yogi Berra, legendary baseball player and manager

Despite its comical undertones, this quote retains an element of insight. Rounding provides a platform from which to view daily operations and learn from these observations.... Dutiful observation often leads to identification of opportunities for improvement....

3. Approachability

"You need to create a safe environment for people to speak up or you're not going to know what's going on." —Alan Mulally, CEO of Ford Motor Company

Being approachable is key to gathering information held by those on the front line. The ability to break down communication barriers will in part determine the overall success of rounding.... Body language and demeanor can have a large impact on how you are perceived.

4. Building Trust

"Rounding has been the key to my success as CEO. How can executives understand the needs of patients, physicians and nurses without interacting with them on a daily basis? When I walk through the hospital, it is a great opportunity to gather information and build trust by listening and responding to concerns. Rounding takes me beyond the paper dashboard so I can get a true pulse on the health of the organization." —Mike Sherrod, CEO of Coliseum Northside Hospital, Macon, GA

Developing relationships with key stakeholders in the organization must be a primary focus of senior leadership. Rounding provides an opportunity for administrators to engage physicians and nurses and build trust. Showing you are committed to providing patients with the best care possible is crucial. Clinicians want to know you are on the same team....

Leader Versus Boss

When I was elected president of my high school service club, my father, a **Green Brain** mechanical engineer, who was founder and president of Lab-Line Instruments, Inc., shared the following anonymous poem with me. This poem often was included in the Lab-Line monthly employee-published *HI-LITER* newsletter. I continue to share the following wise words with others in my **WCIYB?** Programs and in my *BrainBuzz* newsletter.

The Leader

The boss drives group members; the Leader coaches them.
The boss depends upon authority; the Leader on good will.
The boss inspires fear; the Leader inspires enthusiasm.
The boss says, "I will," the Leader says, "We will!"
The boss assigns the tasks; the Leader sets the pace.
The boss says, "Get here on time";
the Leader gets there ahead of time.
The boss fixes the blame for the breakdown;
the Leader fixes the breakdown.
The boss makes work a drudgery; the Leader makes it a game.
The boss says, "Go"; the Leader says, "Let's go!"
The world needs Leaders; but nobody wants a boss!

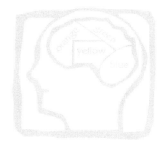

10

YOUR PERSONAL RELATIONSHIP WITH FAMILY MEMBERS AND FRIENDS

You Have a "Personal" Gemstone Personality

As you may recall, you learned the following from Chapter 2: *Recognize Your Professional Strengths and Perspectives*:

- Someone might describe you as a gem because he or she knows something good about you.
- You often use the word *gem* to describe an individual whose Brain Color is esteemed or valued.
- You understand more about the **WCIYB?** approach and will find it easy to think of yourself as a multifaceted gemstone-quality person.
- You can easily connect to the gemstone metaphor visually, emotionally, culturally, and/or historically.
- You will remember that gemologists say that gemstones have their own personalities and are valued most for the brilliance of their colors.
- Just like a gemstone, you will value others and are attracted to the best features of their personalities.

From *What Color Is Your Brain?® When Caring for Patients: An Easy Approach for Understanding Your Personality Type and Your Patient's Perspective.* Published by SLACK Incorporated. Copyright Sheila N. Glazov. http://www.sheilaglazov.com

The current chapter will offer a summary of your personal relationships with your partner, children, family members, and friends. For a more in-depth perspective of those relationships, refer to Chapters 7, 8, 9, and 10 of my original **What Color Is Your Brain?**® book.

Your Best "Personal" Features

A gemstone is faceted to show off its best features. To discover the best features of your personality in your personal life, take your **"Personal" Brain Color Quiz** (presented over the next few pages), and match your **A, B, C, and D TOTALS** to each of the four Brain Color **Personal** Strengths and Perspectives on the **Personal Brain Color Strengths and Perspective** charts.

As you know from scoring the **Health Care Professional Brain Color Quiz** in Chapter 1, the **Personal Brain Color Quiz** is a "No Right or Wrong Answer," easy personality profile that will provide you with a visual tool to analyze your characteristics. This tool is also a method for which to recognize your attributes and abilities in your home or in a community environment, as well as with your partner, children, family members, and friends.

A fellow yogi, Siri LeBaron, sent me (Sheila N. Glazov) the following email message:

> I read your book on my train ride home. I'm a total Blue Brainer. No surprise. I think I have one Orange bit. Then my partner took the quiz and he's a super *Green* Brain, with a couple Orange dashes. Oh, my! We read through a lot of the book and I so amazed with the EASE this has brought to our communication. Like you said, it's an explanation, not an excuse. But that understanding changes so many things. "Green Brain Thing" and "Blue Brain Thing" have already become a frequent part of our "Couple's Talk." So interesting!

The **Personal Brain Color Quiz** also consists of word lists and fill-in-the-blank sentences. The numerical values from this process will give you a synopsis of your personality and a logical ranking of your **Personal** Brain Colors.

Because you have been reading all this new Brain Color information, I trust that you are embracing your new knowledge and are not feeling overwhelmed. The following will help you to refresh your memory and determine your **Personal** Brain Color:

1. Your Brain Colors may be different in your personal life than in your health care professional life.

2. Remember to focus on the **Personal** perspective of your life when reading the descriptive words and sentences.

3. Read all the words across the page before you begin to numerically determine their value.

4. If you think two or more words in a row are of equal value, remember your perspective—it is your **Personal** life. Or, to remind yourself, try the following sentence: "In my personal life, I am _____."

5. You might feel it to be more comfortable and helpful to use "inaccurate" instead of "wrong" and "accurate" instead of "right" when selecting your answers.

6. This is not a "**wanna be**" quiz. It does not determine *who you want to be*; it determines who you *are* at this time in your **Personal** life.

7. If you are reading this with another individual, please do not have him or her help you. The purpose of this quiz is for *you* to confirm your own Brain Color. If the other individual is a family member or friend, he or she might think he or she knows you better than you know yourself. Don't forget—how you see yourself may not be how others see you!

8. Enjoy this fun and informative **Personal** Brain Color quiz; it will be informative and fun!

9. Refer to the charts on pages 112-113 to explore your Brain Color Strengths and Perspective.

Directions

- Read the **four** words and sentences horizontally → across each row on the page.
- Decide which word in each row describes you: *Most* = **4**; *Not as much* = **3**; *Not too much* = **2**; and *Least* = **1**.
- Rank each characteristic in the row across → using 4, 3, 2, and 1 **only once** (i.e., **4** = the **greatest value** and **1** = **least value** to you).
- **Tip:** Read all four choices before numerically ranking your selection.
- After you have completed **all** the rows →, **vertically** add **all** the numbers in **each** of the **four** columns down ↓ to calculate your **TOTALS**.
- Record the **TOTAL** number for your **A**, **B**, **C**, and **D** columns in the appropriate **TOTAL** spaces at the bottom of the page.
- If two of your **TOTALS** are numerically equal, this is *not* unusual.

If you add all of your **TOTALS** together, your **TOTAL** numerical ranking should equal **110**.

The Personal Brain Color Quiz

A	B	C	D
__ Organized	__ Creative	__ Independent	__ Enthusiastic
__ Punctual	__ Communicative	__ Curious	__ Fun loving
__ Detailed	__ Flexible	__ Composed	__ Competitive
__ Responsible	__ Caring	__ Analytical	__ Resourceful
__ Committed	__ Sensitive	__ Contemplative	__ Courageous
__ Thorough	__ Cooperative	__ Technical	__ Energetic
__ Accountable	__ Affectionate	__ Autonomous	__ Adventurous
__ Respectful	__ Authentic	__ Competent	__ Generous
__ Predictable	__ Nurturing	__ Investigative	__ Spontaneous

When making decisions, I like to:

__ Have a plan	__ Talk to others	__ Gather all facts	__ Trust instincts

When interacting with others, I see myself as a:

__ Coach	__ Team player	__ Problem solver	__ Troubleshooter

I am most comfortable and thrive in an environment that supports my sense of:

__ Stability	__ Harmony	__ Privacy	__ Freedom

TOTAL A __	TOTAL B __	TOTAL C __	TOTAL D __

The following items reiterate what you learned previously in Chapter 2: *Recognize Your Professional Strengths and Perspective*s:

1. You may find it helpful to read about your Personal Brain Colors according to their numerical sequence.
2. Read first the **A, B, C, or D TOTALS** that ranked the highest and read last the one you ranked the lowest.
3. You will discover that most of your characteristics are under the descriptions you ranked the **highest**.
4. If two of your **TOTALS** are numerically equal, that is not unusual. It indicates similar **Personal** Strengths and Perspectives in those Brain Colors.
5. It is normal to recognize a **few** of your characteristics in the other Brain Colors Strengths and Perspectives descriptions.
6. The other Strengths and Perspectives descriptions will also offer insight into other people's best features.

Your Best Perspectives

While you were identifying your **Personal** Brain Color Strengths and Perspective, did you think:

- "I can't believe how accurate this was!"
- "I'm a _____Brainer and my partner is a _____ Brainer."
- "My best friend is _____Brainer."
- "Each of my children is a _____Brain Color!"

Personal and Professional Relationships

This book is focused on your **Health Care Professional Brain Colors**. However, it is essential to recognize and understand your personal Brain Color connections that build harmonious relationships with your romantic partner, children, family members, and friends and how those relationships may or may not influence your emotions and behavior in the workplace and with your patients.

Your personal Brain Color attributes can influence your relationship with your patients, their relatives, and friends, and your coworkers. Some Brain Color personalities find it more difficult or easier to deal with the professional aspects of their life than the personal ones.

Having a clear understanding of your best personal Brain Color strengths and perspective is significant for you and is critical for understanding your patients' personal relationship with their family members and friends. This valuable knowledge will help you to recognize and comfortably deal with the diverse Brain Color behaviors of your patients' relatives and friends and will help you know how those behaviors affect the patients' well-being and influence everyone's interaction with one another.

Be the Best of Whatever You Are
If you can't be a pine on the top of the hill,
Be a scrub in the valley, but be
The best little scrub by the side of the rill;
Be a bush if you can't be a tree.
If you can't be a bush be a bit of the grass,
And some highway some happier make;
If you can't be a muskie then just be a bass~
But the liveliest bass in the lake!
We can't all be captains, we've got to be crew,
There's something for all of us here.
There's big work to do and there's lesser to do
And the task we must do is the near.
If you can't be a highway then just be a trail,
If you can't be the sun be a star;
It isn't by size that you win or you fail~
Be the best of whatever you are!
—Douglas Malloch

A—YELLOW BRAIN PERSONAL STRENGTHS AND PERSPECTIVE

PERSONAL STYLE: Regimented

ROMANTIC STYLE: Loyal

PARENTING STYLE: Strict disciplinarian

WITH OTHERS: I inform them of "my" rules

I'M PHYSICALLY ATTENTIVE: At appropriate times

I SHOW LOVE BY: Taking care of my loved ones

EMOTIONALLY I NEED TO: Be in control

FINANCIAL APPROACH: Save money

I ENCOURAGE: Respectfulness

STRESS FACTOR: Irresponsibility

I RELAX: Only if everything is finished

C—GREEN BRAIN PERSONAL STRENGTHS AND PERSPECTIVE

PERSONAL STYLE: I don't interfere

ROMANTIC STYLE: Reserved

PARENTING STYLE: Be independent

WITH OTHERS: I'm not overly complimentary

I'M PHYSICALLY ATTENTIVE: When no one is watching

I SHOW LOVE BY: Actions, not words

EMOTIONALLY I NEED TO: Be selective

FINANCIAL APPROACH: Systematize money

I ENCOURAGE: Self-sufficiency

STRESS FACTOR: Others meddling in my business

I RELAX: By myself

B—BLUE BRAIN PERSONAL STRENGTHS AND PERSPECTIVE

PERSONAL STYLE: Thoughtful

ROMANTIC STYLE: Affectionate

PARENTING STYLE: Helpful

WITH OTHERS: I am a genuine communicator

I'M PHYSICALLY ATTENTIVE: As much as possible

I SHOW LOVE WITH: Hugs and kisses

EMOTIONALLY I NEED TO: Feel appreciated

FINANCIAL APPROACH: Share money

I ENCOURAGE: Flexibility

STRESS FACTOR: Overextending myself for others

I RELAX: With friends, family, and pets

D—ORANGE BRAIN PERSONAL STRENGTHS AND PERSPECTIVE

PERSONAL STYLE: Optimistic

ROMANTIC STYLE: Spontaneous

PARENTING STYLE: Open minded and fraternal

WITH OTHERS: I let them be themselves

I'M PHYSICALLY ATTENTIVE: Anywhere, any time

I SHOW LOVE BY: Giving surprises and gifts

EMOTIONALLY I NEED TO: Feel uninhibited

FINANCIAL APPROACH: Spend money

I ENCOURAGE: Taking risks

STRESS FACTOR: Others telling me what to do

I RELAX: With physical activity

Personal Versus Professional Behavior

Yellow Brainers' personal relationship style is disciplined and dedicated. They can transfer and apply those personal attributes to their workplace by being "**Rependable**." The word "**Rependable**" was created by a 5th grader named Eric, who told me, "I am a Rependable Yellow Brainer, which means I am responsible, respectful, accountable, and dependable." Yellow Brainers are capable of adapting their behavior to focus on their patients and their workplace tasks, and they do not let their emotions "get the best of them" because that would not be the "right thing to do."

Blue Brainers' personal relationship style is thoughtful and devoted. They transfer and apply those personal attributes to their workplace by showing their compassion and sincere listening skills to their patients. However, they often find it difficult to separate their personal life from their professional life, and they must be careful not to let their feelings interfere with their patient care and workplace tasks.

Green Brainers' personal relationship style is to be objective and not interfere. They transfer and apply those personal attributes to their workplace by judiciously controlling their emotions. It is easy for them to put their personal life "in a box" or "on the shelf." They are capable of not having their personal life or perspective affect how they care for their patients and handle their workplace tasks.

Orange Brainers' personal relationship style is easy going and optimistic. They transfer and apply those personal attributes by focusing on the "in the moment" situations. They are capable of quickly turning their emotional switch on or off, depending on the circumstances. They handle whatever must be done for their patients or their workplace tasks by doing the most urgent first.

Your "AAAA" Partner Relationship Road Map

In the relationship with your partner, a variety of personal characteristics and talents attracts us to this individual. Think of your "**AAAA**" **Partner Relationship** journey as a solution to dilemmas that dampen successful relationships. The following is your **AAAA Partner Relationship** road map:

1. Recognize what **Attracted** you to each other.
2. Understand why different idiosyncrasies have become an **Annoyance**.
3. **Accept** your loved one for who he or she is and what he or she values, even if his or her ideas differ from yours.
4. **Appreciate** why you fell in love with each other to keep the romantic spark that ignited your positive attraction from fizzling into a negative reaction!

Positive Attractions

Yellow Brainers are romantically attracted to:

- Other Yellow Brainers who respect their personal routines.
- Orange Brainers who contribute adventure to their routine.
- Blue Brainers who cooperate with their projects.
- Green Brainers who provide structured systems for them.

Blue Brainers are romantically attracted to:

- Other Blue Brainers who reciprocate their show of affection.
- Yellow Brainers who respect their feelings.
- Green Brainers who give them a logical perspective.
- Orange Brainers who encourage their creativity.

Green Brainers are romantically attracted to:
- Other Green Brainers who also value solitude.
- Blue Brainers who are thoughtful.
- Yellow Brainers who keep precise records.
- Orange Brainers who seize opportunities.

Orange Brainers are romantically attracted to:
- Other Orange Brainers who will join in their fun.
- Blue Brainers who encourage their enthusiasm.
- Green Brainers who help them to calculate risk.
- Yellow Brainers who plan their activities.

Negative Reactions

We are often drawn to another individual because he or she has the personality traits and talents that we do not have or we would like to have. Remember, what first attracted you in your romantic relationship might later annoy you and cause a negative reaction.

Yellow Brainers become annoyed when:
- Other Yellow Brainers become too domineering.
- Blue Brainers act like scatterbrains.
- Green Brainers do not give them all the details.
- Orange Brainers do not respect their rules.

Blue Brainers become annoyed when:
- Yellow Brainers restrain their creativity.
- Other Blue Brainers drain them with their extra drama.
- Green Brainers dismiss their feelings.
- Orange Brainers exhaust their enthusiasm.

Green Brainers become annoyed when:

- Yellow Brainers intrude on their solitude.
- Blue Brainers talk too much.
- Other Green Brainers insinuate that they know more.
- Orange Brainers "fire" before they take "ready and aim."

Orange Brainers become annoyed when:

- Yellow Brainers restrict their fun.
- Blue Brainers coddle them.
- Green Brainers criticize them.
- Other Orange Brainers change their minds too often.

Your Family Vacation

Do you feel like you are spending your vacation with the soap opera cast members of **General Hospital** or the models from *FamilyFun* magazine? Either would be an unforgettable opportunity to examine your Brain Color relationships. Some facts about each Brain Color on a family vacation are as follows:

Yellow Brainers arrange for well-planned family vacations. Their family vacations are scheduled each year at the same time and at the same place, such as a summer cottage or resort. They love being the tour guide and do their homework ahead of time, planning the entire trip.

Blue Brainers love reunions with family members, close friends, classmates, and neighbors. They also love nature trips. Vacations are opportunities to share time with everyone they love. They also would not think of excluding their pets, as they are part of the family, and will take them along by staying in accommodations that are advertised as being pet friendly.

Green Brainers prefer to travel on their own or with a small group of individuals who share the same interest in what they are going to experience. They enjoy investigatory or educational tours of significant historic events, museums, and ruins of ancient civilizations or locations where they can acquire instructive information.

Orange Brainers love spontaneity and variety during their family vacations. They find unfamiliar or exotic places and meeting new people exciting. Exciting sports trips are at the top of their list. A spur-of-the-moment trip or a short weekend getaway is the perfect escape from the boredom of their daily routine.

Friends to the Rescue

The following tips will help to enhance your relationship and cooperation with friends:

- If you would like to ask a friend with whom you drive to work to help you prepare for a surprise dinner party, but you know she is **Orange**, always late, and never arrives on time, say, "I'd like you to be **Yellow** and arrive at my home promptly at six o'clock to assist with the preparation of my surprise dinner party. I know I can depend on you!"

- If you need a **Yellow** friend to give you a hand cleaning the dinner dishes, do an errand for you because you are have the flu and cannot get out of bed, or make some telephone calls for your favorite charity fundraising benefit, say, "I need you to be **Blue** and help me with the dinner dishes," "help me out by running some errands for me while I am sick," or "support my favorite charity fundraiser by making some telephone calls for me, please!"

- If you are **Blue** and having a problem getting your children to do their homework, you cannot figure out how to operate a new computer program you recently installed, or you cannot figure out how to logically deal with a problem, tell a friend, "I could really use your **Green Brain** to explain the new system on my computer" or "I am sure you can help me figure out this problem so I will not be an emotional wreck."

- Your **Orange** college friends are enthusiastic about planning your next reunion. However, if you are **Green** and grumpy because of a problem you cannot solve with a coworker, say, "Okay, I can be **Orange** and not be a party pooper while you are planning our reunion. I am sorry I have been so cranky and spoiling your fun with complaints about my coworkers."

An Understanding Friend

We often consider our family members as our friends and our friends as our family members. In the following poem, "Friendship," Bessie P. Owens expressed how joyful it is to be understood, share a meaningful bond, and receive irreplaceable acceptance:

A smile and cheerful greeting
from someone on life's way;
A handclasp warm and tender,
how it brightens up the day!
Just to feel that understanding
when our hope's about to end,
And life is sad and weary...
Oh, the joy to have a friend.

Comparing Children's, Students', and Adults' Brain Color Statistics

The statistics shown in **Figure 10-1** on the following page and in the sections that follow, were assembeld from my research projects and programs. The data will demonstrate the unique comparison between children's, students', and adults' Brain Colors. This information will also help you maintain more harmonious relationships with the individuals in your personal life, those you care for, and those with whom you interact in your health care workplace.

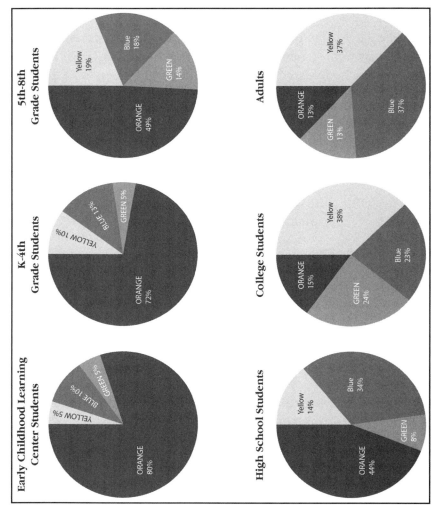

Figure 10-1. Brain Color statistics for children, students, and adults.

Brain Development

Notice that the percentage (**Figure 10-1**) of Orange (frontal lobe) for the early learning and elementary school students is twice that of the Yellow (temporal lobe) for adults. That contrast can significantly influence your relationship with young children.

In her book, *Mapping the Mind*, author Rita Carter stated:

> A nucleus called the reticular formation, for example, which plays a major role in maintaining attention, usually only becomes fully myelinated at or after puberty, which is why prepubescent children have a short attention span. There are approximately 86 billion neurons in the brain. The neurons that connect the cells in the frontal lobe do not become fully myelinated [myelin is a sheath of white substance that acts as insulation, allowing electricity to flow swiftly and directly to sections of the brain] until full adulthood. This is one reason, perhaps, why younger adults are more emotional and impulsive than those who are older.

The percentage contrast of brain development shown in the pie chart of the early childhood learning center through eighth grades (**Figure 10-1**) explains the frustration between Yellow Brain adults and Orange Brain children. However, the contrast between a Yellow Brain adult and an Orange Brain high school student is less (**Figure 10-1**) because children of high school age have a more developed frontal lobe. The frontal lobe usually does not completely develop until an individual is between the ages of 25 and 30.

Notice the small percentage of high school students who are Green Brainers (**Figure 10-1**). High school is usually the time that teenagers learn to drive a car. This small percentage of logic and problem solving explains why insurance policies are so expensive for teenager drivers!

YELLOW BRAIN CHILDREN'S/STUDENTS' STRENGTHS AND PERSPECTIVE

I LIKE TO: Be careful

I AM: A leader

AT SCHOOL: I assist the teacher

I LEARN BEST: When I'm prepared

AT HOME: I follow the rules

WITH FRIENDS: I make plans to be together

I NEED: Exact instructions

I LIKE TO READ: History and biographies

I AM UNCOMFORTABLE: Without structure

WHEN SICK AND FEARFUL: I worry

TO ENCOURAGE ME, SAY: "I'm proud of you."

 GREEN BRAIN CHILDREN'S/STUDENTS' STRENGTHS AND PERSPECTIVE

I LIKE TO: Solve problems

I AM: A computer wiz

AT SCHOOL: I like to quietly work alone

I LEARN BEST: Using books and computers

AT HOME: I don't show my emotions

WITH FRIENDS: I'm a loner, not in the crowd

I NEED: Time to figure things out

I LIKE TO READ: Mysteries and science fiction

I AM UNCOMFORTABLE: With too much noise

WHEN SICK AND FEARFUL: I don't like to talk

TO ENCOURAGE ME, SAY: "I think you're smart."

**BLUE BRAIN CHILDREN'S/STUDENTS'
STRENGTHS AND PERSPECTIVE**

I LIKE TO: Honestly talk about my feelings

I AM: An artist

AT SCHOOL: I help my friends

I LEARN BEST: When visual aids are used

AT HOME: I like to be shown lots of love

WITH FRIENDS: I am a good listener

I NEED: Hugs or high fives

I LIKE TO READ: Fantasy and animals stories

I AM UNCOMFORTABLE: If no one listens to me

WHEN SICK AND FEARFUL: I am hypersensitive

TO ENCOURAGE ME, SAY: "I love/like you."

 **ORANGE BRAIN CHILDREN'S/STUDENTS'
STRENGTHS AND PERSPECTIVE**

I LIKE TO: Perform

I AM: An athlete

AT SCHOOL: I like to "do" instead of "listen"

I LEARN BEST: With hands-on activities

AT HOME: I like to "do my own thing"

WITH FRIENDS: I like to play games and sports

I NEED: Fun

I LIKE TO READ: Adventure and sports stories

I AM UNCOMFORTABLE: With too many rules

WHEN SICK AND FEARFUL: I can be defiant

TO ENCOURAGE ME, SAY: "You're fun to be with."

The Psychology Fair

I facilitated a Brain Color study at the student psychology fair at Fremd High School, Palatine, Illinois. The following percentages represent the 194 students who participated in the research project:

- 43% **Orange**: Are highly impulsive and action-oriented (percentage is opposite that of adults).

- 31% **Blue**: Have a high level of desire to please others and gain peer approval (percentage is similar to that of adults).

- 15% **Yellow**: The sense of responsibility and accountability for the choices they make is unusually low (percentage is opposite that of adults).

- 11% **Green**: Level of logical reasoning about the consequences for their actions is extremely low (percentage is similar to adults).

The Teenage Brain

The student psychology fair statistics indicated in the previous section demonstrate why living and working with a teenager can be tumultuous, even if the adult and teenager are of the same Brain Color.

- A Yellow Brain teenager wants to have more control than the adult's over his or her life and thinks, "Times have changed and your rules are old fashioned."

- A Blue Brain teenager thinks, "You can't possibly understand my feelings and what I'm going through!"

- A Green Brain teenager thinks he or she is smarter than the adult. When our eldest son was a teenager, we hung a "If You Want to Know Everything, Ask a Teenager!" sign over his bedroom door.

- An Orange Brain teenager would be in total agreement with Katharine Hepburn, who said: "If you obey all the rules, you miss all the fun."

I encourage you to use **WCIYB?** to help you survive your child's teenage years or until your child becomes a young adult and realizes that you are no longer the enemy, that you have a brain, and that they can build and maintain a harmonious relationship with you!

Children's and Students' Brain Color Differences

The previous Brain Color charts and statistics will help to improve your understanding of what makes your young children, preteen, and teenage patients zig while other youngsters zag. Knowing what makes your patients tick and recognizing their Brain Color strengths and perspective will help you build a collaborative relationship with and determine how to motivate each youngster in a health care and/ or home environment.

Fun Breaking Down the Pieces

by Kristine E. Yung, OTR/L

I had the experience of working with a Green Brain young boy who had absolutely no interest in writing or coloring. He was more interested in how an object worked or how the toy was put together. On a weekly basis, I would try to find a manner in which I could get him excited about the opportunities of writing and being able to express his great ideas.

I tried to imagine the task from his perspective when a light bulb turned on. We then transformed the letters into animals or machines or cars. We would draw the basic letter, then rotate the paper and transform the letter into another object. So, the letter "B" became the base of a truck, with the two humps forming the wheels. Then, we had to think of another letter to place on the truck to help us with forming the freight that we were going to haul. He chose the letter "H," which he then transformed into two boxes filled with toys.

It became exciting and fun for him to write the letters, and his goal was to draw a picture with every letter. It was the opening that I needed to help him to learn the skill of writing. I have kept his drawing of the letters and how we transformed them into various items, such as a snake, lion, plane, or building. His strength of wanting to break items apart to determine how they were put together led me to the exciting path of breaking letters into pieces and discovering his creativity.

Element of Fun

In the movie *Mary Poppins*, Julie Andrews tells Michael and Jane Banks, "In every job that must be done, there is an element of fun. You find the fun and—SNAP—the job's a game!"

Using the Brain Color approach will add an element of fun to your personal relationships with your partner, family members, friends, and children of all ages.

According to author Richelle Mead, "There are little gems all around us that can hold glimmers of inspiration." I believe that our Brain Color talents, personality traits, and perspectives are those little gems that inspire us to build loving, respectful, joyful, and healthy personal bonds with our partners, family members, and friends.

In this chapter, you determined your **Personal** Brain Colors, recognized the best qualities of your family members and friends, and learned how to enhance and encourage your personal relationships!

*"When we seek to discover the best in others, we somehow
bring out the best in ourselves."*
—William Arthur Ward

SECTION II: BRAIN COLOR PROFESSIONAL AND PERSONAL CONNECTIONS SUMMARY

Brain Color Connections	Yellow Brainers	Blue Brainers	Green Brainers	Orange Brainers
Connection with adult patients	Explain details about their care	Be an attentive listener	Ask "yes" or "no" precise questions	Acknowledge their loss of freedom
Connection to pediatric patients	Understand their feelings of insecurity	Let them cry if they need to	Do not treat them like a "baby"	Use play to help them feel more comfortable
Connection and cooperation with coworkers	A "well done" pat on the back	Truthfulness and no gossip	Acknowledge their innovative ideas	Getting results quickly
Coworkers' frustrations	Disorder and tardiness	Apathy and conflict	Redundancy and intrusions	Negativity and waiting
Connection with management and agencies	Realistic approach with management and agency representatives	Considerate of management and agency representatives	Not talkative; gives facts to management and agency representatives	Helpful troubleshooters with management and agency representatives

(continued)

From *What Color Is Your Brain?® When Caring for Patients: An Easy Approach for Understanding Your Personality Type and Your Patient's Perspective.* Published by SLACK Incorporated. Copyright Sheila N. Glazov. http://www.sheilaglazov.com

SECTION II: BRAIN COLOR PROFESSIONAL AND PERSONAL CONNECTIONS SUMMARY (continued)

Brain Color Connections	Yellow Brainers	Blue Brainers	Green Brainers	Orange Brainers
Partner's positive attraction	Respect his or her personal routines	Reciprocate his or her show of affection	Value his or her solitude	Join in his or her fun
Partner's negative reaction	Becoming too domineering	Restrain his or her creativity	Interrupt his or her solitude	Restrict his or her fun
Family members' and friends' needs	Schedules and dedication	Conversations and compassion	Solitude and "no meddling"	Freedom and optimism
Children need	Exact instructions	Hugs or high fives	Time to figure things out	Fun
Children are uncomfortable	Without structure	When no on listens to them	With too much noise	"Do" instead of "listen"
Children who are sick and fearful	I worry	I am hypersensitive	I don't like to talk	I can be defiant
To encourage a child, say:	"I'm proud of you."	"I love/like you."	"I think you're smart."	"You're fun to be with."

From *What Color Is Your Brain?® When Caring for Patients: An Easy Approach for Understanding Your Personality Type and Your Patient's Perspective.* Published by SLACK Incorporated. Copyright Sheila N. Glazov. http://www.sheilaglazov.com

SECTION III

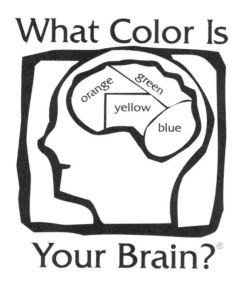

BRAIN COLOR
COMMUNICATION AND
COLLABORATION

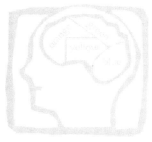

11

LISTEN AND SPEAK FLUENT BRAIN COLOR

Color is a universal language.
Carl Jung, renowned for his four basic personality types said,
"Colors are the mother tongue of the subconscious."

Brain Color as a Second Language

When people travel to another country, they often attempt to learn the native language or a few helpful phrases. However, you do not have to leave your workplace or home to become fluent in Brain Color. Children often become fluent in Brain Color faster than do adults. However, I am confident that you can learn to speak fluent Brain Color and make it your second language as thousands of adults and children have done over the past 20 years.

One day, while I was shopping and speaking with the store owner, who speaks fluent Brain Color, another shopper suddenly interrupted, saying, "You're the Brain Color lady aren't you? You're Sheila Glazov!"

"Yes, I am," I responded.

"I remember you because of your Brain Colors. I am an Orange Brainer," she said. "We met while I was working in

From *What Color Is Your Brain?® When Caring for Patients:*
An Easy Approach for Understanding Your
Personality Type and Your Patient's Perspective.
Published by SLACK Incorporated.
Copyright Sheila N. Glazov. http://www.sheilaglazov.com

the children's clothing store where you had an author signing for your children's book, ***Princess Shayna's Invisible Visible Gift.***"

We had not seen each other for almost 10 years! I was amazed and delighted that she still spoke fluent Brain Color.

Pay Attention

Pay attention to your conversations with others, as people will reveal their Brain Color by how they converse:

- **Yellow Brainers** will ask about your home or the community in which you live or your career.
- **Blue Brainers** will ask about your family, friends, and pets.
- **Green Brainers** will ask about where you went to school, what level of education you have, or the books you like to read.
- **Orange Brainers** will ask about your hobbies or favorite vacation.

You can always use these topics of conversation when you are introduced to someone you do not know and want to get to know better. If you want to utilize your Green Brain and do not want to ask personal Blue Brain questions; you can engage your Orange Brain and ask people what they like to do for fun.

Speaking and Understanding Fluent Brain Color

To fluently speak and understand Brain Color, it is essential to recognize and determine an individual's Brain Color and communication style by the specific words they select when speaking with you.

The chart on page 135 will help you to determine and understand an individual's Brain Color and communication style by the specific words they select when speaking with you:

Brain Color Communication Styles Comments

Brain Color Comment	Yellow Brain	Blue Brain	Green Brain	Orange Brain
"I admire your ability to be…"	Organized	Cooperative	Objective	Courageous
"Thank you for…"	Being prompt	Listening	Solving the problem	Your generosity
"I appreciate your sense of…"	Responsibility	Compassion	Fairness	Adventure
"I don't understand why he or she is so…"	Self-righteous	Idealistic	Condescending	Impulsive
"I am uncomfortable when he or she is…"	Controlling	Sensitive	Uncommunicative	Procrastinating
"I don't know why he or she is being…"	Inflexible	Emotional	Insensitive	Immature

From *What Color Is Your Brain?® When Caring for Patients: An Easy Approach for Understanding Your Personality Type and Your Patient's Perspective.* Published by SLACK Incorporated. Copyright Sheila N. Glazov. http://www.sheilaglazov.com

How Do You Communicate?

Whether people use a letter, invitation, telephone call, email, blog post, text message, Facebook post, or tweet, each person will communicate consciously or subconsciously from their Brain Color perspective.

- **Yellow Brainers** "have to" communicate and be responsible: "I will be attending the professional conference."
- **Blue Brainers** "love to" communicate and share with others: "We are going to be grandparents!"
- **Green Brainers** "need to" communicate for a purpose: "Our office requires a patient's medical history."
- **Orange Brainers** "want to" communicate something exciting: "Hurrah, I just got a promotion!"

Please Tell Me More …. And

Depending on the circumstances, each Brain Color individual will or will not tell you more about a situation, himself or herself, or other people.

- **Yellow Brainers** will tell you more information because they feel responsible about informing you and making sure you have all the correct details.
- **Blue Brainers** will tell you more because they enjoy sharing information, and they feel they are helping others when they tell them what they know about the circumstances.
- **Green Brainers** do not want to tell you more because they think you do not need to know. This makes sense to them because if they would not be interested, why should you?
- **Orange Brainers** will tell you more because they are excited about the information, and will tell you how to achieve the desired results or how to initiate some type of change.

If you would like more information from another Brain Color, you can reply with the following:

- "Yes, that is correct, and I would like to know more details about…" to a **Yellow Brainer**
- "I appreciate your sharing of that information, and it would be helpful to know more about…" to a **Blue Brainer**
- "You are telling me all the basic information, but I also need to know more precise specifics about…" to a **Green Brainer**
- "Wow, that is exciting information, and it would be terrific to know more about…" to an **Orange Brainer**

Make It Easier Communication Clues

The following Brain Color Communication Clues make it easier to communicate in color and fluently speak Brain Color with each Brain Color personality.

Communication With Yellow Brainers

- Be polite and punctual.
- Respect their personal values of organization and rules.
- Stay on track.
- Tell them all the details.
- Encourage them to talk about their achievements.

Communication With Blue Brainers

- Show you are sincerely listening.
- Respect their emotions.
- Use stories to explain your point of view.
- Connect with them personally.
- Encourage them to talk about their family.

Communication With Green Brainers

- Do *not* make small talk.
- Respect their privacy.

- Be brief, but informative.
- Give them lots of statistics and data.
- Encourage them to talk about their knowledge, not yours.

Communication With Orange Brainers

- Be direct.
- Respect their spontaneity.
- Make your point quickly.
- Give them the results, not facts and figures.
- Encourage them to talk about their hobbies or vacations.

What Are You Selling?

Because you are a health care professional, you may not think of yourself as a sales professional. However, everyone experiences times when they must sell themselves to gain a promotion or to make a patient feel more comfortable or sell their ideas to make changes in departmental or office procedures and/or skills to improve patient care. The following are examples to help you recognize the Brain Colors of the individuals with whom you are interacting:

- **Yellow Brainers** will tell you they have to look at their calendar to determine if they can schedule a time to meet with you.
- **Blue Brainers** will talk to you about their relationship with your colleague, friend, or family member who referred you to them, and is likely to say, "I'd be happy to help you out."
- **Green Brainers** may not answer their phone because they do not like to talk on the phone—they prefer a text or email. If they do answer, tell them you a researching a solution to a problem that will create more efficiency in their medical facility or in patient care.
- **Orange Brainers** will say they are eager to meet with you and ask, "How soon can we get together?"

Sincerely Listening Skills

If you are selling yourself, your ideas, or a product, you also must demonstrate sincere listening skills. The following are Sincere Listening Skills that Raymond Kayal, Jr., CEO of Newslink Group, LLC, graciously shared with me when I facilitated programs for his executive team and airport store team members:

10 Clues for Sincere Listening

1. Clear you mind of preconceived ideas.
2. Discipline or force yourself to sincerely listen.
3. Be objective, not emotional.
4. *Hear* and pay attention what you are being told.
5. Recognize that there is something *critically important* in what is being said.
6. Identify the direction the speaker wants to go in the conversation.
7. Be aware to fish out and capture all the potential golden nugget ideas.
8. Articulate your perspective.
9. Be open to a different point of view.
10. Think, process, and concentrate on what you are listening to and don't busy your brain with a premature answer.

Are You Listening?

If you sincerely listen when others communicate, you hear them consistently, and often unconsciously, tell you the color of their brain. It is easy to refine your listening skills or have fun by politely eavesdropping whenever possible.

- **Yellow Brainers** use words such as **"should," "would,"** and/or **"have to"** when they are talking about themselves or others.
- **Blue Brainers** tell you how they **"love"** or **"feel"** about something or someone.

- **Green Brainers** respond with, "I'll have to **think** about that."
- **Orange Brainers** say, "That sounds like **fun**. What are we waiting for? Let's do it!

Show and Tell

by Jill Cook, RN, CDE

I recently had a patient who had been sent to us because her HbA1c [glycated hemoglobin] was more than 12% for more than 1 year, and she was taking a large amount of insulin. When I was doing her intake, I noticed that what she was telling me and what her blood sugars were did not make sense. I asked her to demonstrate how she was giving herself insulin. She could tell me the proper steps, but it was easy to see the problem when she actually gave insulin to herself. Instead of pushing the pen plunger down, she thought it was easier to wind it down, thus not getting any insulin. So, for more than 1 year, she thought she was giving herself 60 units of mixed insulin before each meal, but she was not giving any!

She now is well controlled on 10 units of insulin before each meal. Sometimes it just takes listening and watching what the patient is doing to help them.

Improve Your Communication and Listening Skills

There is always room for improvement to enhance your communication and listening skills, which will increase harmony with your patients, colleagues, and supervisors. The following Brain Color tips may help to improve your communication and listening skills:

YELLOW BRAINERS

- Need to be more open minded.
- Ask others to put their thoughts in a written document.
- Call for a group meeting so that everyone involved receives the correct information.

BLUE BRAINERS

- Do not become *too* emotional and take things to heart.
- Talk less and listen more.
- Speak to be more assertive.
- Use your authenticity to speak up and offer candid comments.

GREEN BRAINERS

- Be patient.
- Do not be thinking of what you are going to say next instead of actively listening.
- Use your natural abilities to remain calm.

ORANGE BRAINERS

- Pay attention.
- Do not have side conversations with others.
- Use natural skills to negotiate or troubleshoot.

Life and Death Situations

by Nancy Maruyama, RN, BSN

I always wanted to be a nurse. I found that I really enjoyed working in a hospital, caring for patients with chronic illnesses or recovering from surgical procedures. As a Blue Brainer, I expected that I would always work in a similar setting. However, life doesn't always go the way we plan. As it turns out, my real calling is working with the bereaved. What's that saying? "Takes one to know one?" Guess so.

Overnight, I went from a first-time mom of a 4-½ month old son, to a bereaved parent. My first child, my only son, Brendan, was a victim of SIDS (Sudden Infant Death Syndrome). He died at the baby-sitter's on a Friday morning 5 weeks after I returned to working at the clinic of a large teaching hospital. If not for Karen, another SIDS mom who was also a nurse, I am not sure I would have survived those first few years after my son's death.

The local SIDS organization, now called Sudden Infant Death Services (SIDS) of Illinois, Inc., reached out to my husband and me and offered comfort and the emotional resources with which to go on living. Two years after Brendan's death, I gave birth to my first *subsequent child**, a beautiful daughter who we named Caitlin. Twenty-three months later, our second beautiful daughter, Jennifer, was born. Around this time, I found my true calling as a nurse.

In 1998, the Executive Director of SIDS of Illinois, Inc. wrote and received a grant, allowing me to provide "grief sensitivity" education to police departments in Illinois. The goal of the education was to help law enforcement officers understand how empathy for newly bereaved parents in acute settings is mutually beneficial for both the parents and the investigation. Report after report came to me from the bereaved parents I was working with. Aside from the obvious, I kept hearing from parents that they were being accused of harming or even killing their babies! In almost every case, it was eventually determined that the parent(s) had done nothing to purposely cause the deaths of their babies.

Around this time, I met Tom, a wonderful retired Illinois state trooper, who agreed to let me have 60 minutes of speaking time during his trainings of juvenile officers and child abuse investigators. What stood out so obviously was that the officers were Green Brainers. It was not that they did not possess empathy, but they were protecting themselves from the emotional pain and fear of losing a child. Parents are not meant to bury their children. That is just not the way it is supposed to be!

What I learned from the police officers is that they cannot be effective at their jobs if they do not keep their emotional guards up. Many of the officers had infants or grandchildren of their own and said if they left themselves open to this vulnerability that they would absolutely lose their minds. There is something akin to comfort about the task of "being a Green Brainer and logically following the Yellow Brain checklist" to the officers who respond to these calls; so often they do their best to not let themselves be Blue and feel their emotions.

There is also the fear that death will knock at their doors. This is not an unreasonable fear. Nurses can have these same fears when they provide care to the bereaved parents as well. They just respond differently to the situation. By nature, nurses tend to be Blue Brain *nurturers*. Law enforcement officers tend to be Green Brain problem solvers. Both disciplines have the need to help, to fix, and to solve.

After I became aware of the different response processes, it was easier for me to comprehend how people's Brain Colors affect the way they handle difficult situations. It allowed me to further understand why newly bereaved parents, nurses, and police officers react as they do when responding to infant death.

Subsequent child. The subsequent child is new and unique—not a replacement for the child who died.

For many bereaved parents, there is often great emphasis placed on the term *subsequent child*. Those children are also referred to as *rainbow babies* because, after a time of tears and great mourning, the clouds of grief begin to lift and the sun once again begins to shine and begins of a time of healing for the bereaved parents.

Effective Communication = Health Literacy

According to The Joint Commission, which is an independent, not-for-profit organization that accredits and certifies more than 20,500 health care organizations and programs in the United States, effective communication is a cornerstone of patient safety.

The following excerpt is the conclusion in the white paper **What Did the Doctor Say?: Improving Health Literacy to Protect Patient Safety** (http://www.jointcommission.org/assets/1/18/improving_health_literacy.pdf). The article is not only applicable in the United States and in English-speaking countries, it is relevant in any health care facility around the world:

The communications gap between the abilities of ordinary citizens, and especially those with low health literacy or low English proficiency, and the skills required to comprehend typical health care information must be narrowed. Hundreds of studies have revealed that the skills required to understand and use health care-related communications far exceed the abilities of the average person. The high rate of adverse events related to communication breakdowns, now widely recognized, is also widely believed to be unacceptable. The amelioration of medical error and adverse events must begin with creating cultures of safety and quality... must be designed to protect the patient's safety and invite the patient's participation in his or her care.... that will permit patients to receive more time, attention, education and understanding of their conditions and their care.

No matter what language is spoken in the hospital, health clinic, or medical office that you work, it is critical for you to understand how each Brain Color patient deals with health care literacy to prevent mistakes and to efficiently communicate safe health care information and helpful instructions.

- **Yellow Brain Patients** may be too proud to say that they cannot read or do not understand what the health care professional is telling them. Their lack of communication can be caused by embarrassment.

- **Blue Brain Patients** do not want to be labeled as a "problem patient." They do not want to cause any type of disruption and will be agreeable, even if they do not understand what is being said.

- **Green Brain Patients** are uncomfortable asking questions because they do not want to admit they cannot read, and they feel foolish admitting that they do not understand what they are being told.

- **Orange Brain Patients** think that they can figure out how to handle the medical situation and do not have to pay attention and follow the health care professional's instructions that they do not understand.

Strategies for Effective Communications With Other Brain Colors

Brain Colors	Yellow Brainer Strategies	Blue Brainer Strategies	Green Brainer Strategies	Orange Brainer Strategies
Yellow Brainers	Detailed instructions Have a plan Respect decisions	Be encouraging Let them talk Respect emotions	Have a logical plan No "yes" or "no" questions Respect explanations	Don't be bossy Value their energy Be open-minded
Blue Brainers	Clear expectations Be prepared Take notes	Be cooperative Sincerely listen Validate feelings	Don't be emotional No excessive talking Do your homework	Share ideas Express feelings Enjoy activities
Green Brainers	Step-by-step plan Specific instructions Respect their rules	Show appreciation Brainstorm Value creativity	Only necessary facts Time to process Ask for facts	Explain incentives Show end results Be patient
Orange Brainers	Be prompt Be respectful Be polite	Praise creativity Offer help Talk with them	Give all the facts Be resourceful Slow down	Competitive ideas Time for fun No meetings

From *What Color Is Your Brain?® When Caring for Patients: An Easy Approach for Understanding Your Personality Type and Your Patient's Perspective.* Published by SLACK Incorporated. Copyright Sheila N. Glazov. http://www.sheilaglazov.com

Make It Easier

Using your Brain Color knowledge and skills makes it easier to:

- Recognize the point of view of your patients and their family members.
- Sincerely listen to your patients' and their advocates' perspective.
- Recognize health literacy to improve patient safety.
- Communicate your health care professional perspective.
- Sell yourself, your ideas, and your health care expertise.
- Improve your communication and listening skills with patients, their family members, and coworkers.
- Deal with challenging, including life-threatening and death, situations.

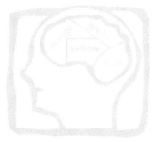

BUILD RAPPORT AND COLLABORATE WITH OTHERS

Do We Have as Much Sense as the Geese?

The following story was written by Dr. Harry Clarke Noyes. I have adapted it and use it in all my **WCIYB?** team building programs. I think you will find it insightful and beneficial.

When you look up and notice geese flying, you may wonder why they fly in a "V" formation. You might be interested in knowing just what scientists have discovered about why geese fly that way. It has been discovered that as each bird flaps its wings, it creates uplift for the bird immediately following it. By flying in a "V" formation, the entire flock will add at least 71% greater flying range than if each bird were to fly on its own. Whenever a goose falls out of formation, it suddenly feels the drag and resistance of trying to go it alone, and it quickly returns to the formation, taking advantage of the uplifting power of the bird flying immediately in front of it.

Basic Truth #1: People who share a common direction and/ or sense of community can arrive at their destination or goal remarkably quicker and easier because they will be traveling on the thrust, TRUST*, and TRUSTWORTHINESS* of one another.

Basic Truth #2: If we have as much sense as a goose, we will continue in a formation with those who are headed in the same direction as we are.

When the lead goose tires, he will rotate to the back and allow another goose to fly lead position.

Basic Truth #3: Whether with people or geese flying, it will pay to take turns doing the hard jobs.

Geese will honk from behind to encourage those up front to keep up their speed.

Basic Truth #4: We want to encourage those up front, but at the same time we need to be careful what we say when we "HONK" at them from behind.

When a goose is sick or wounded and falls out of formation, two geese will fall out of formation and follow it down to help and to protect it. They will remain with it until it is either able to fly or until it dies. They will then launch out on their own, or with another formation, to catch up with their own group.

Final Truth: If we have as much sense as the geese, we will support one another—similar to the way the geese support each other!

*TRUST: A strong sense of openness and sharing of ideas and feelings.

*TRUSTWORTHY: The ability to accept others and their contributions, to support, recognize, and affirm others' strengths and capabilities and exhibit cooperative and honest intentions.

Brain Color Connection Clues

The following Brain Color Connection Clues will help you to establish rapport with patients and build exceptional patient care:

 YELLOW BRAINERS

- Use a diplomatic tone.
- Use a formal approach.
- Make the patients feel secure.
- Understand the patients' sense of commitment.
- Acknowledge the patients' *follow the rules* motto.

 BLUE BRAINERS

- Use a cooperative tone.
- Use a friendly approach.
- Make the patients feel appreciated.
- Understand the patients' sensitivity.
- Acknowledge the patients' *we can help each other* motto.

 GREEN BRAINERS

- Use an informative tone.
- Use an academic approach.
- Value the patients' intelligence.
- Understand the patients' sense of brevity.
- Acknowledge the patients' *think it through thoroughly* motto.

 ORANGE BRAINERS

- Use an encouraging tone.
- Use a relaxed approach.
- Acknowledge the patients' informal style.
- Understand the patients' nontraditional"sense of style.
- Acknowledge the patients' *let's go for it!* motto.

Building Rapport
With Trust and Trustworthiness

In 1985, our eldest son was 15 years old and was diagnosed with T1D (Type 1 diabetes). We were living in Mammoth Lakes, California, which was a small ski resort community in the Sierra Nevada Mountains. Joshua was diagnosed on the Friday after Thanksgiving, and I immediately began my Green Brain research to find care and knowledge for our son and myself.

My first call was to our friend and physician, Dr. David Green, who informed me about a diabetes clinic in Sparks, Nevada, which was a 3- to 6-hour drive, depending on the weather and road conditions through the mountains. The clinic was also offering a 5-day diabetes class beginning on Monday.

By Sunday afternoon, Joshua's glucose level and my emotions began to stabilize. We were prepared for our journey to the diabetes clinic. Joshua was filled with food and insulin; the car was filled with gas, a blanket, a shovel, and a snow broom, as well as snacks, soda pop, and juice. I was filled with determination, even though I was scared to death that I might do something wrong to harm Joshua.

I was relieved to make the trip in 3 hours without encountering a blinding snowstorm, 70-mile per hour winds, or cattle grazing in the middle of a mountain road. We arrived safely at Sparks Family Hospital, registered for the clinic, and then settled into the empty pediatric ward for the night.

On Monday morning, we met Joshua's amazing health care team. Sally and Sue were his diabetes nurse educators and Libby was his registered dietitian and diabetes educator. We spent 5 days—from 9 o'clock until 4 o'clock—in the clinic classroom, learning everything we need to know about T1D. It was easy and comfortable for Joshua and me to build a rapport with Joshua's diabetes team. Sally and Sue were the humorous tag-team instructors, who made sure we understood every T1D concept and procedure. Libby was our easy-going and fun-loving nutritional coach, who made sure we understood the new dietary information about carbohydrates, proteins, and fats (the food exchange system was being phased out) and how critical it was to balance and keep a record of Joshua's meals, physical activities, and insulin in his log book.

After 5 days of intensive training, Joshua and I graduated from the diabetes class. As we drove home, we were less afraid and more knowledgeable about T1D management and nutrition. We learned to **trust** our team and our own judgment because of the strong sense of openness and sharing of ideas and feelings. Joshua and I built a **trustworthy** rapport with each other and our team by accepting one another's contributions; supporting, recognizing, and affirming our capabilities; and cooperating with honest intentions. Sue, Sally, and Libby continued to be Joshua's diabetes team until our family moved to Chicago in 1989. Joshua and I remain grateful to and have fond memories of his dynamic diabetes health care trio!

Trust is the glue of life.
It's the most essential ingredient in effective communication.
It's the foundational principle that holds all relationships.
—Stephen Covey

"I Do Not Want To Be Touched!"

by Dr. Randy J. Horning, DC

Lisa, a young woman who had been abused by her father, was referred to me because she was suffering from neck pain and severe headaches. During her first visit, she told me, "I want to be fixed, BUT I DO NOT WANT TO BE TOUCHED!"

As a Blue Brainer, I understood her discomfort and concern and did not touch her during her range of motion and eye and ear examinations. Afterwards, I encouraged her to have a massage to relieve her pain. Lisa finally agreed, as long as her friend was in the room, and she wanted to be fully clothed while under the sheet on the massage table. Lisa had several massage sessions, but, her condition did not change much; however, she did become more comfortable with the female massage therapist's gentle touch. We continued to do range of motion exercises to increase her mobility, and, eventually, I was able to convince her to have electric muscle stimulation on her back while she wore a tank top that exposed her back.

I was finally able to build a level of trust by talking to Lisa and demonstrating my sincere concern for her health and well-being. Eventually, I was able to perform very gentle traction on her neck. After several traction sessions, Lisa felt comfortable enough for me give her an adjustment. After two adjustment appointments, her neck pain was gone and her headaches disappeared. It took 3 months of patience, trust building, and developing a sense of safety when she was touched before Lisa was no longer in pain and was feeling well!

Build Rapport and Enhance Collaboration

The following examples can help you adjust your Brain Color behavior to build rapport and increase collaboration with patients, their family members and advocates, and your coworkers and other individuals with whom you interact every day.

Yellow Brainers need to be flexible to change and more considerate of other people's beliefs, plans, and/or expectations.

Blue Brainers need to be less sensitive to criticism and more mindful of other people's communication styles and emotions.

Green Brainers need to be more aware of other people's concerns and more cognizant of other people's solutions to a problem.

Orange Brainers need to be more focused on the "team" instead of on "me" and more observant of other people's methods to achieve the desired results.

A Collaborative Approach

by Ellen Sherman, PhD

My work and approach as a therapist is called "collaborative." From my therapeutic perspective, collaboration means finding solutions from both within and without the individual's perspective. This approach requires that one understands and integrates the solutions from many sources. In health care, the health care worker brings his or her perspective to the issue, and the individuals, families, and physicians each have another perspective—the interaction of all of these contribute to the outcome.

An example of this approach comes from my own doctoral dissertation. My research focused on an individual and her family interacting with health care professionals. The patient had a chronic condition that caused her to be unable to work, and she was in constant pain. The patient's collaborative team included physicians and surgeons, her parents, her siblings, and me. She honored me by allowing access to all of these people, who were trying to influence her medical decisions. Her difficult journey and its resulting solution became the basis of my research and writing.

Finding the patient's perspective was the first step in the process, which took place over several weeks through conversation. When I asked to speak to her family, whom she deemed unsupportive, there was some hesitation. She decided that because so much time was spent constructing her story, she would allow me access to her "team," including her family and the medical specialists.

Utilizing our collaboration and how the patient perceived both the problem and the solution, my task was made easier by understanding her thinking. My research also included how people in other cultures conceptualize illness. With this co-creation, her family finally stopped standing in the way of her view of treatment and her perception of her future with this condition. It also appealed to the medical professionals because when they listened to her story, they realized that there was more than one approach to her situation.

Twenty years later, this patient, who simply wished to be heard and understood, still suffers from the chronic condition. However, she has built a functioning existence, manages her medications, and lives independently, using friends and family for support. Her type of personality required the understanding of a collaborative team of medical professionals, alongside her family and friends.

Certainly, other health care professionals' conversations and collaborations have contributed to a new approach that seems to fit with other thinkers—the individual's perspective must be taken into account in medical settings. It seems that the "collaborative" time has come.

A Health Care Clinic Connection Game

I find it amusing to observe and try to decode people's Brain Colors while I wait in my physician's, dentist's, or chiropractor's office for my appointments. In today's world, with people's challenging schedules, waiting for health care services has become more complicated and stressful. However, you can make it "color filled" and entertaining.

Do you remember the car traveling games, Car Colors, Cow Count, and License Plate Search? Now, you can play the **Health Care Clinic Connection Game**. Use your Blue Brain to imagine that you are visiting family members for a holiday celebration or visiting a friend for a vacation. Your recurring cough has worsened and you agree to see a physician, but the office is closed. You do not want to go to the hospital emergency department; instead, you drive find yourself to a crowded neighborhood health care clinic. To pass the time, you inquisitively observe your fellow patients and entertain yourself by thinking about the possible Brain Color connections you would have with them.

Health Care Clinic Connection Game Guidelines

- Keep an open mind. (*Under different circumstances, you may not want to make a connection.*)
- Fill in the blanks with the appropriate Brain Colors.
- Write each of the Brain Colors only once in each Connection section.

- Have fun!
- Remember—it's just a game!
- Confirm your answers at the end of this chapter.

The Riveted Reader

You cannot help noticing the man tethered to his laptop. He is definitely not a winning candidate for the *Gentleman's Quarterly* magazine cover model contest. A coffee cup, doughnut shop bag, and *The Wall Street Journal* are a jumble of fossils beneath his chair. His oversized, sun-dried attaché case, pregnant with technical manuals for various computers, is slumped in the seat between you.

If you began to choke on the protein bar you brought with you, he would not even notice. However, if in your distress, you flung yourself over his mountain of reading material, you would capture his attention. He would administer an effective Heimlich maneuver, and return to his work unfazed.

Your Brain Color Connection

The Riveted Reader is a _____ Brainer. You connect with him because you are a:

1. _____ Brainer and laugh because his jumble of fossils reminds you of your office.
2. _____ Brainer and you have similar reading material in your briefcase.
3. _____ Brainer and he reminds you of your favorite uncle.
4. _____ Brainer and you should tell him that the flight is boarding and the gate has been changed.

Mrs. Fran Friendly

You have signed the check-in list and are waiting your turn. The woman sitting next to you is wearing a pastel-flowered, gardening-themed sweater, with matching pink watering can earrings. A charm bracelet, with pictures of her children dressed in their baseball uniforms, adorns her wrist.

She asks if you have been a patient at this clinic before. You tell her it is your first time at the clinic, and she responds with a recitation of her entire family's medical history. In only a few minutes, you know each of her family members by name, including the pets. Then she offers an apology and says, "I've been such a chatterbox, I haven't given you an opportunity to tell me about yourself."

Your Brain Color Connection

Ms. Fran Friendly is a _____ Brainer. You connect with her because you are a:

1. _____ Brainer and a freelance sports writer compiling research for an article about soccer moms.

2. _____ Brainer and feel like you and a long-lost friend were reunited.

3. _____ Brainer and well-mannered. However, you are **not** interested in sharing your vital statistics and family history, nor will you exchange email addresses and telephone numbers to stay in touch.

4. _____ Brainer and amused by the reruns of "This Is Your Life, Fran Friendly."

A Crocodile Cowboy Biker

On the way to an empty seat, you nearly stumble over a pair of crocodile, silver-tipped cowboy boots. An eccentric-looking gentleman apologizes, stands up, tips his cowboy hat, and invites you to sit down next to him. He is wearing a toffee-colored, deerskin-fringed jacket and cowboy hat trimmed with spotted snakeskin, a bleached lizard jaw, and delicate quail feathers.

As you sit down, he tells you, "I'm in town visiting my former neighbors and I began feel'n kind of poorly. I didn't want to spoil the fun we were having, but they insisted that I come to clinic and get checked out." Then he regales you with his life stories as an attorney, a real estate developer, a private pilot, and a Harley motorcycle rider.

Your Brain Color Connection

The Crocodile Cowboy Biker is a _____ Brainer. You connect with him because you are a:

1. _____ Brainer and accept a silver-embossed business card because he could be a valuable business connection in the future.

2. _____ Brainer who also rides a Harley motorcycle and wants to purchase a 1970s muscle car.

3. _____ Brainer and knows he is a quick course in entrepreneurship, which could be useful after 25 years in corporate America.

4. _____ Brainer and are inspired and entertained by his stories.

Martha Stewart of the Midwest

You sit down next to a woman who looks like a senior model for a Ralph Lauren line of clothing. She is impeccably dressed; her cordovan loafers have a military gloss, and she is reading *The Clutter Busting Handbook*. She properly covers her mouth with an ironed, monogrammed linen handkerchief when she coughs.

You decide to ask if she would like a drink of water from the water dispenser in the waiting room. She gratefully says, "Yes, thank you, I just spent 3 weeks helping my youngest daughter and her family move into their new home. I think I overdid it and overstayed my welcome."

Your Brain Color Connection

The Martha Stewart of the Midwest is a _____ Brainer. You connect with her because you are a:

1. _____ Brainer and find her a pleasure. You tell her that her family is fortunate to have such a talented mother and grandmother.

2. _____ Brainer and intrigued by her wealth of knowledge, which sounds like a "moving day" version of the *Gettysburg Address*.

3. _____ Brainer and know you need to learn more about her Extreme Nanny Techniques for Disciplining Toddlers and Teenagers.

4. _____ Brainer and are ready to take an advanced placement class in Helpful Household Hints for the Working Woman.

Now, you can enjoy playing the **Health Care Clinic Connection Game** wherever you are—in a health care clinic or doctor's office, a holiday cocktail party, a commuter train station, a business conference "meet 'n greet," or while you are traveling. You will find your Brain Color observations and connections with others entertaining instead of aggravating.

Build Rapport and Collaboration With Courtesy

Courtesy
I am a little thing with a big meaning.
I help everybody.
I unlock doors, open hearts, and dispel prejudice.
I create friendships and good will.
I inspire respect and admiration.
Everybody loves me.
I bore no one,
I violate no law.
I cost nothing.
Many have praised me,
None have condemned me.
I am pleasing to those of high and low degree.
I am useful every moment of the day.
I am Courtesy!
—Anonymous

Your Brain Color Connection Answers

- The Riveted Reader is a Green Brainer. You connect with him because you are:
  1. Orange
  2. Green
  3. Blue
  4. Yellow

- Ms. Fran Friendly is a Blue Brainer. You connect with her because you are:
  1. Green
  2. Blue
  3. Yellow
  4. Orange

- The Crocodile Cowboy Biker is an Orange Brainer. You connect with him because you are:
  1. Green
  2. Orange
  3. Yellow
  4. Blue

- The Martha Stewart of the Midwest is a Yellow Brainer. You connect with her because you are:
  1. Blue
  2. Green
  3. Orange
  4. Yellow

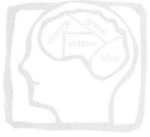

OFFER EXCEPTIONAL PATIENT CARE

Excellent Professional Behavior = Excellent Patient Care

I designed the **What Color Is Your Brain?® Behaviors of Excellence** chart when I had the Yellow Brain privilege and Orange Brain pleasure of collaborating with Matthew L. Primack, PT, DPT, MBA during a Leadership Development Institute at Advocate Condell Medical Center. The Behaviors of Excellence is also referred to as the BOE and is a corporate Advocate Condell Medical Group initiative.

The BOE help patients to feel cared for because they experience extraordinary service and quality care.

- When health care professionals implement the BOE, they know that their patients are receiving superb care.

- When health care team members utilize the BOE, they feel valued and know that their contributions in their health care facility are consistent, respected, and make a difference for their patients and their coworkers.

What Color Is Your Brain?® and Behaviors of Excellence

Behavior of Excellence	Yellow Brain	Blue Brain	Green Brain	Orange Brain
Be responsive	Speak politely	Listen sincerely	Acknowledge need for privacy	Accept rules
Be respectful	Value promptness	Value communication	Value information	Value spontaneity
Be professional	Follow policies	Encourage cooperation	Demonstrate competency	Negotiate skillfully
Be accountable	Keep detailed records	Keep promises	Keep accurate research	Keep seeking best reults
Be collaborative	Organize ideas	Share ideas	Analyze ideas	Promote ideas

From *What Color Is Your Brain?® When Caring for Patients: An Easy Approach for Understanding Your Personality Type and Your Patient's Perspective*. Published by SLACK Incorporated. Copyright Sheila N. Glazov. http://www.sheilaglazov.com

Offering Excellent Patient Care

When dealing with sensitive issues, such as fear, denial, and confusion, it is essential to know how to offer excellent patient care according to the Brain Colors of the patient and his or her health care professional.

 Yellow Brain Health Care Professionals Offer Excellent Care to:

- **Yellow Brain** patients by understanding that they are upset about not being in control of their care.
- **Blue Brain** patients by being friendly and dependable.
- **Green Brain** patients by respectfully answering questions about their health condition.
- **Orange Brain** patients by explaining why it is important to follow hospital policies.

 Blue Brain Health Care Professionals Offer Excellent Care to:

- **Yellow Brain** patients by listening when they want to discuss the details of their care.
- **Blue Brain** patients by letting them talk about their concerns for their family and/or pets.
- **Green Brain** patients by not making small talk with them.
- **Orange Brain** patients by encouraging their physical activity and rehabilitation.

 Green Brain Health Care Professionals Offer Excellent Care to:

- **Yellow Brain** patients by preparing them with appropriate information before a medical procedure.
- **Blue Brain** patients by letting them talk and ask questions about their health care plan.
- **Green Brain** patients by logically explaining how their medical strategies will solve their health problems.

- **Orange Brain** patients by telling them to comply with the health plan to recover faster.

 Orange Brain Health Care Professionals Offer Excellent Care to:

- **Yellow Brain** patients by understanding their discomfort about others being in charge.

- **Blue Brain** patients by showing them empathy when they have to "let off steam."

- **Green Brain** patients by having patience regarding all of their requests and questions.

- **Orange Brain** patients by acknowledging their frustration while being confined.

Military Tool Box for Mental Health

by Marylyn Harris, RN, MSN, MBA
Psychiatric nurse practitioner and addictions nurse

I began my 35-year nursing career as an Army medic (MOS 91B), which is a military occupational speciality, also known as a combat medic. My true story is an example of how health care professionals and the patients we care for can benefit from the "Military Tool Box of Skills," which was gleaned from my service in the United States Army from 1981 to 1992 as an Army nurse, an x-ray technician, a decorated war veteran, a disabled veteran, a veterans' advocate, a psychiatric nurse practitioner, and an addictions nurse.

MISSION: In 1998, I received an assignment to *locate*, *engage*, and *connect* a Harris County (Texas) chronically mentally ill patient to existing services. In my role as the *Homeless Outreach Nurse Practitioner* at the Mental Health Authority, this case was distinctively unique, compared with the traditional cases that I was usually assigned.

INTELLIGENCE: I was informed that the patient was a schizophrenic woman who, over the years, cost Harris County more than $1,000,000. Reportedly, she was challenging to locate, was difficult to engage, was noncompliant with medications, and refused to be treated by health care providers. The patient's previous medical records revealed a three-decade (30 year) history of mental illness, excessive inpatient admissions (> 30 per year), and gross noncompliance with medical treatment regimens and advice.

TEAM BUILDING: My agency partner on this case was a licensed social worker. She was an expert in working with the most challenging chronically mentally ill cases. She was a member of the agency's *Assertive Community Treatment (ACT) Team*.

OPPS PLAN: Together, my agency partner and I devised a preliminary strategy to locate, engage, and reconnect the patient to medical and psychiatric services to improve her quality of life and reduce the county's mental health financial expenditures significantly. On our first attempt to locate Miss "Cissy" (not her real name), we were moderately successful.

HAZARDOUS DUTY: We were given an address for Miss Cissy, which was in a low-income neighborhood in Houston. Upon pulling up to the address, we noticed a huge glaring hole in the side of the house. The home did not look fit for human habitation, and no one answered the doorbell when we rang it. Someone a couple of doors down began hollering at us, *"You looking for Miss Cissy?"*

INFORMANT: As our heads turned to follow the noise, the person shouted, *"Well, she ain't there!"* We returned to our car and slowly drove down the street toward "the voice." The gentleman informed us that he was a "neighbor" of Miss Cissy and that she was at the church up the street. He told us that in the mornings, she helps to serve breakfast to the elderly at the local church.

Feeling a sense of accomplishment, we thanked the neighbor, and proceeded to locate the church to which he directed us. Upon arriving, the church was locked. We decided that we would return to the neighborhood early the next morning and go directly to the church.

The next morning was 90-plus degrees in Houston. When my colleague and I arrived at the church, the church staff members were hesitant to share information with us about Miss Cissy. Miss Cissy was not at the church serving breakfast to the older adults that morning. We were able to confirm that she did "volunteer" often at the facility. However, the church staff would not confirm nor deny that she would be back at the church the next day, or ever.

MISSION FOCUSED: We decided to comb the neighborhood that morning and try to locate Miss Cissy. We had no physical description of her and no "script" of what to say to her should we be fortunate enough to locate her. As we rode through the neighbor-hood, we were taken aback by the obvious poverty of the residents and the condition of the dwellings they called home.

RECONNAISSANCE: After turning a corner, we found ourselves driving behind a woman wearing tight, neon orange Spandex pants. Her body was as shapely as her walk was brisk. She wore a long, brown, curly wig—the type that Diana Ross wore when The Supremes topped the music billboard charts. Miss Cissy noticed us before we noticed her.

"That's a preeeeety car," she said.

Instantly and instinctively, I knew that she was Miss Cissy!

I said, *"Hi,"* as I was on the side of the candy apple red Mustang convertible closest to her.

"Do you need a ride?" I asked.

She said, *"Uh, OK, I am a little tired of walking this morning; it's HOT."*

Interestingly, it was the red convertible that was instrumental in connecting us to Miss Cissy.

INTERVENTION: While we were driving, we explained to Miss Cissy who we were and the community services that we provided.

RAPPORT BUILDING: Initially, she refused to discuss her illness or anything about her personal life. As we continued to build a rap-port with her, we showed up in the mornings and took her to the church for her "volunteer job," as she called it. Miss Cissy loved to arrive at the door being chauffeured in the red convertible Mustang.

Ironically, it was the church staff who shared their concerns about Miss Cissy after the church activities. We were informed that Ms. Cissy *"prostituted"* at night *"to make ends meet."* After all, she was quite fit and beautiful for a 70-year-old woman. Miss Cissy had the shape of a 35-year-old and did not hesitate to flaunt it.

Over the course of the several months that we worked with Miss Cissy, she began to trust us. I learned so much about love, survival, and mental illness. She has remained one of my favorite patients.

GOAL ORIENTED: Eventually, Miss Cissy began to allow me to con-duct mental status exams and mini-physical assessments. My goals were to assess her mental and physical status and connect her to community resources to meet her needs.

RESOURCES: Each time I visited, I brought bag lunches and appropriate treats to Miss Cissy and her 90-plus-year-old mother, who lived with her in their dilapidated house. I also offered a plethora of resources available through our agency and our strategic community partner organizations.

Eventually, Miss Cissy allowed me to medicate her in her living room with her prescribed intramuscular antipsychotic deconate medication. I felt assured, knowing that Miss Cissy was safe and would have relief from the recurrent negative symptoms of long-term, untreated paranoid schizophrenia.

Over time, as I continually assessed her symptoms, I saw improvement in Miss Cissy's condition, poverty of thoughts, and recurrent hallucinations. I began to talk to her about coming into our clinic to see the doctor (psychiatrist). After several weeks, Miss Cissy was ready for us to transport her to an appointment with the doctor at the clinic visit.

SUCCESS: We worked exclusively with Miss Cissy for 1 year. During that time period, she was never hospitalized, jailed, or had any negative incidents in her personal life. We saved Harris County tens of thousands of dollars by intervening successfully with Miss Cissy. This patient was managed successfully on her antipsychotic medications, her medical needs were addressed, and she was connected with community resources for food, shelter, and clothing (and more). As far as we know, she ceased prostitution-type activities and re-engaged with her family members and community groups (church). Being supported and case managed in a way she had never before experienced, Miss Cissy thrived!

Until...

ADVOCATE: Many months later, a young man who was visibly suffering with psychotic symptoms came into our clinic. I pleaded with the agency medical staff on site at the clinic to see this young man, and he was told to return to the clinic the next day. I was told that I could telephone the county mental health constables to commit the man to the psychiatric hospital. However, upon returning to the clinic lobby, the young man was gone.

The next day, a Houston television "Breaking News Flash" revealed that a mentally ill homeless man allegedly robbed a pregnant woman of her purse at a shopping center near downtown. He allegedly then traveled downtown and stole a briefcase from an attorney leaving court. This young man was unarmed. His activities were allegedly witnessed by an "off-duty judge," who followed the young man eight blocks up a one-way downtown street and shot him dead in broad daylight. His dead body lay uncovered on a Houston sidewalk for more than 2 hours.

This young man was the patient I pleaded with our psychiatrist to see the day before in the clinic where I worked. The psychiatrist had refused. The young man was now dead. I was informed when I returned to work the next week that this homeless, mentally ill young man was Miss Cissy's son.

LEADERSHIP: Although I had met Miss Cissy's son only briefly in the clinic a few days before, I asked the ACT Team if I could go to see Miss Cissy, talk with her about her son's untimely death, assess how she was doing, and determine whether there was anything she needed or anything we could do for her.

On many levels, I feared that she would relapse after hearing this news. When I reached her, it was apparent to me that no one had informed her of her son's death. I took a very deep breath and told her that her son had been killed.

I will never forget the look in her eyes and the words she said to me when I told her that her son had been murdered.

Having no children at the time and never having lost a child, I was not prepared for the avalanche of emotion that I experienced with Miss Cissy on that day. I supported her in the best ways I knew how by remembering my wartime experiences and numerous deaths, of comforting loved ones of war casualties, and of supporting health care professionals cope with the stress of war.

I utilized my nursing skills and knowledge of the grieving process and evolution of loss. I practiced Irvin Yalom's *"genuineness and thereness"* tenets and focused on the *"here and now"* with Miss Cissy. I assisted her in getting to the place where her son's body was being kept, acquiring additional information, and making burial arrangements. I followed up with her after his death, continued to assess her needs, and made appropriate referrals. Sometimes, I just went to her house and sat quietly with her. It was a very challenging situation.

I knew then, and I know now, that this was a distinctively unique case that changed my nursing practice and my life. I am eternally committed to be an ultimately skilled and compassionate health care professional. Miss Cissy and her entire family (mother and son) were mentally ill. Thousands of mentally ill persons "quietly" exist in cities across America. The mentally ill have *rights!* They have the same constitutional rights as the rest of us—the right to life, liberty, and the pursuit of happiness. The community that Miss Cissy lived in failed her, and the state of Texas failed her! She never should have been allowed to exist as she was when we encountered her—untreated, unmedicated, living in deplorable conditions, and prostituting for money to survive. Her community and those in it contributed significantly to perpetuating her state of mental illness.

Many times, we ignore mental illness and call it everything except what it is—*mental illness*. Even as health care professionals, we see mentally ill people struggling and we hesitate to intervene. Many of the mentally ill are in our own families and neighborhoods and impact each of our lives! Mental illness touches every community and every race, ethnicity, and socioeconomic status. As health care professionals, we can become involved in our workplace and community organizations that help mentally ill citizens to successfully reintegrate into society. *Then we all will benefit!*

Patient Comfort

Excellent patient care includes the unique way each individual relates to his or her patient from his or her Brain Color that makes the patient, as well as the Health Care Professional, feel comfortable. The following are ways in which the Brain Colors create feelings of comfort:

YELLOW BRAINERS

- Discuss their plan of care.
- Introduce themselves and ask patients what they prefer to be called.
- Make sure patients feel safe in an unfamiliar environment.
- Are polite and prompt.

BLUE BRAINERS

- Intuitively assess patients' feelings and needs.
- Offer therapeutic touch.
- Show genuine concern for patients.
- Genuinely ask patients how they are feeling.

GREEN BRAINERS

- Let patients know they are capable.
- Ask patients why they have come to the health care office, clinic, or hospital.
- Speak calmly.
- Tell patients exactly what is going to be happening to them.

ORANGE BRAINERS

- Let patients know you are putting yourself in their shoes.
- Respond to patients' needs as quickly as possible.
- Tell patients a joke or a funny story.
- Be cheerful when appropriate.

Golda's Veterinarian

I know from my own personal experiences that **WCIYB?** is helpful when you have to make critical health decisions about the people and the pets you love. Blue Brainers do not distinguish between their loved ones, whether they have two legs or four legs, fur, feathers, or fins. They all are family members!

Over the years, our family has loved and cared for many cats and dogs. However, my beloved companion was our Golden Retriever/Newfoundland/Labrador, Golda My Dear. When I noticed Golda had an unusual cough, I made an appointment for her at our family veterinarian. After several x-rays and extensive laboratory work, Dr. Hinkle compassionately said, *"Golda has lung cancer."*

The diagnosis shoved my heart through a paper shredder. Then, Dr. Hinkle, our Green/Blue Brain veterinarian, who fluently spoke Brain Color, said, *"Rainbow Lady, I know this is terribly hard for you; you are so Blue. Go home and think about how you want to care for Golda."*

His comforting words helped me to navigate the road home. I knew I had to remain calm. I could not become hysterical and cause an accident that would endanger Golda and me or someone else. By the time we arrived home, I had shifted my Blue to Green. I commenced my research, encouraged myself to be resourceful, and strategized a hospice plan for Golda.

After 2 weeks of home hospice care to help Golda be as comfortable as possible, I realized my husband and I had to make that final appointment with Dr. Hinkle. It was an excruciating decision. However, knowing I had done my best to give Golda the care she needed, I had peace in my heart and reconciliation in my mind.

Because of the exceptional patient care that I gave Golda and that Dr. Hinkle offered to both of us, the challenging experience reinforced an invaluable lesson: No matter what your Brain Color, you can purposely shift to another Brain Color to care for your loved ones; solve even the most difficult, heart-wrenching problems; and make the most arduous and appropriate decisions.

Improving Patient Satisfaction

When an individual, department, health care office, or hospital discovers that they need to refocus and improve patient satisfaction, they need to consider how each Brain Color personality will respond to the problems and solutions. The following are examples of how the Brain Colors respond to such problems and solutions:

 YELLOW BRAINERS
- Implement an effective action plan.
- Hold staff accountable.

- Prepare for retraining.
- Prefer to have the process developed, written down, and scheduled.

BLUE BRAINERS

- Share test results.
- Ask other staff members for suggestions.
- Create visual charts to show improvement options.
- Review patients' point of views.

GREEN BRAINERS

- Analyze metrics.
- Track staff performance.
- Identify barriers.
- Develop spreadsheets.

ORANGE BRAINERS

- Recognize those who are performing well.
- Role-play positive and negative issues.
- Point out complaints.
- Encourage staff by offering rewards.

Tender Loving Care for Patients and Their Families

by MaryAnne Kolker, RN, DN

I respectfully refer to all of my patients as Mr., Miss, or Mrs. I feel it is essential to treat each patient as an equal and not as an individual who is disabled. I assist my patients with their total care—from bathing, dressing, and combing their hair to eating their meals. I have an Orange Brain sense of humor and enjoy teasing the veterans, almost as much as the veterans enjoy teasing me. My husband, Charles, who is a veteran, and I often travel to see our grandchildren. Upon my return to the VA, my patients enjoy teasing me about where I have been and how much they missed me.

Sometimes my patients and I become silly, and I threatens to put ribbons in their hair, dance around their beds, or eat all the stale bread they are saving to feed the ducks in the pond at the VA. Several of my patients cannot speak, but I have learned to read their responses to my questions. One of my patients was a painter before he was injured and lost his sight. Now, he and I enjoy talking about different painting techniques. Sometimes I will sit and listen to the veterans share their stories or tell each other jokes.

One time per month, Charles and I join other volunteers at an Operation Helping Hand dinner for injured veterans and their families. Operation Helping Hand is a project of the Military Officers Association of America (MOAA), which is an organization that helps families of wounded veterans stay with their loved ones while the veterans are undergoing medical treatment. Everything for monthly stays is donated, including rental cars, cell phones, gasoline coupons, entertainment tickets, and food gift certificates. The MOAA provides any comfort or recreation item that will make the families' stay with their loved ones more enjoyable, as well as providing checks for the purchase of needed items. Last, but not least, goody bags and flowers are given to the veterans' families to let them know they are appreciated and help them remember that the volunteeres enjoyed offering them our **Tender Loving Care**!

Do Your Best for Your Patients and Their Families

*"Live your life so that any hour you will be
able to shake hands with yourself
and try to accomplish at least
one thing worthwhile each day.
Then when your nights come,
you will be able to pull up the covers
and say to yourself,
'I have done my best.'"*
—F. Collis Wildman

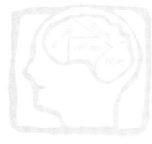

RECOGNIZE AND DEAL WITH BULLY BEHAVIOR

The *Merriam Webster's Collegiate Dictionary*, 11th edition, definitions of *bully* are:

1. Good fellow, fine chap, 2. A blustering, browbeating fellow; one cruel to others weaker than himself, 3. Jovial, dashing, good, or gallant.

Sadly, we hear or read more about the second definition than the others; "school yard" bullies are now joined by an increasing number of "workplace" and "cyber" bullies.

"Nurses Bury Their Young!"

by Sharon M. Weinstein, MS, CRNI, RN, FACW, FAAN

Nurses bury their young! This is a statement that has been repeated from one generation of nurses to the next, and it appears as relevant now as it did when I first entered nursing school many, many years ago.

Why do we do it? Why do we not respect the next generation of nurse leaders who will probably be taking care of us someday? Is it because we were bullied ourselves as students and then as new staff nurses? Is that a reflection of power and control and the Yellow Brain Color? Is it because we had to stand at attention in years past when the nursing supervisor entered the nurses' station

From *What Color Is Your Brain?® When Caring for Patients: An Easy Approach for Understanding Your Personality Type and Your Patient's Perspective.* Published by SLACK Incorporated.
Copyright Sheila N. Glazov. http://www.sheilaglazov.com

and we had to be on our "best behavior?" Now, I am really dating myself.

Because of nursing's fundamental roots as a caring profession, it is difficult to imagine that nurses may not be as respectful to one another and members of the interdisciplinary team as they are to patients.

There is no doubt that the new health care landscape involves disruptive behavior. In health care, disruptive behavior can have negative impacts on safety and patient care outcomes. This is not news! Patients and families assume that doctors and nurses are genuine partners in communication and will work effectively to meet their needs. Yet, bully behavior problems that occur at many health care organizations include yelling, making degrading comments, eye rolling, and refusal to work together.

Bully Behavior Increases as Self-Esteem Decreases

Bully behavior increases as a child's or adult's level of self-esteem decreases. If an individual feels esteemed, he or she would not physically, emotionally, or sexually abuse another person, thus making the other person feel badly about himself or herself. This type of "Shadowed" behavior, when taken to an extreme level, becomes abusive bully behavior.

Bullying and other forms of aggressive behaviors that begin in childhood continue into adulthood if proper intervention is not provided.

We often read or hear about disturbing and, too often, fatal bullying behavior in schools or on the Internet. But, how often do news outlets print or broadcast stories about bully behavior in the workplace, especially a health care facility, where people expect expert and compassionate care?

Workplace bullying is a repeated and unhealthy mistreatment of one or more individuals by one or more perpetrators. Such behavior can include verbal abuse, offensive behaviors, and nonverbal actions, which can be threatening, humiliating, or intimidating. Workplace bullying is a form of sabotage that interferes with critical tasks that need to be accomplished in a health care office or facility.

What Does Bully Behavior Look Like?

The following are 10 examples of bully behavior that can be directed at coworkers, employees, and even patients, their advocates, and family members:

- Excluding or isolating
- Berating or targeting another person in front of others
- Falsely accusing or embarrassing
- Creating unattainable expectations
- Administering extreme disciplinary actions
- Gossiping or rumor mongering
- Taking inappropriate credit or not giving credit where it is due
- Making insulting comments or engaging in negative behavior about others' personality traits or personal life
- Intimidating others
- Coaxing or intimidating others to participate in the bully behavior

Bully Behavior Definitions

The four definitions of individuals involved in bully behavior are:

1. **The Bully:** The aggressor.
2. **The Bullied:** One (an adult or child) who is harassed at work, home, school, or in his or her community.
3. **The Baiter:** One who torments, teases, or goads to provoke a reaction.
4. **The Bystander:** One who does not get involved out of fear or indifference.

Brain Color Bullies

The descriptions of each Brain Color Bully Behavior are as follows:

- **Yellow Brain Bullies:** Must demonstrate they are in charge of a situation or relationship.
- **Blue Brain Bullies:** Engage in passive–aggressive behavior to make other people feel badly.
- **Green Brain Bullies:** Intimidate others with their sense of superior intelligence.
- **Orange Brain Bullies:** Physically dominate others with their size and/or strength.

Brain Color Reactions to Bully Behavior

The descriptions of each Brain Color's reactions to Bully Behavior are as follows:

- **Yellow Brainers** feel bullied when they are forced by others to make a decision without having time to prepare a plan.
- **Blue Brainers** feel bullied and intimidated if someone makes fun of the efforts they make to comfort and encourage others.
- **Green Brainers** think they are being bullied and treated as an outcast when others tease them for being a perfectionist, a "nerd," or a "geek."
- **Orange Brainers** feel bullied when someone uses his or her authority to make them abide by their rigid or unreasonable rules.

Redirecting Bully Behavior

Redirecting the bully behavior might be easier said than done because of the hierarchy in the health care workplace, which the bully uses against his or her victim. The following are examples of how each Brain Color individual can redirect and respond to bully behavior:

- **Yellow Brainers** find a responsible decision-making authorities and notify him or her about the rude or inappropriate bully behavior they experienced.

- **Blue Brainers** need to share their abusive experience with others they feel are trustworthy and capable of obtaining the help they need to put an end to the bully behavior.

- **Green Brainers** will attempt to solve the problem themselves. They can also privately relate the bully behavior to someone they think is competent to assist them, without calling attention to themselves.

- **Orange Brainers'** first reaction is to redirect and deter the bully behavior with a physical response. However, they need to restrain themselves from starting or being part of a fistfight or wresting match.

Brain Color Bully Behavior

The Brain Color Bully Behavior chart on page 180 provides examples of coworkers, patients, family members, individuals in management positions, or agency representatives who exhibit uncooperative, inappropriate, unrealistic, and/or negative behavior that can be considered bully behavior.

Brain Color Bully Behavior

Brain Color Bully Behavior	Yellow Brainers	Blue Brainers	Green Brainers	Orange Brainers
Negative Behavior	Realize they do not have all the details	Do not take their actions personally	Ignore the bully	Let negativity roll off their backs
Uncooperative Behavior	Offer detailed examples and information	Validate their feelings, allow them to vent	Ask direct questions and offer facts	Offer humor and/or positive perspectives
Argumentative Behavior	Calmly explain in detail all of the lessons to be learned	Listen and then ask them how they are feeling	Explain logical cause and consequences	Let them know you understand how they feel
Unrealistic Behavior or Requests	Speak directly: "Let's look at A, B, and C."	"I am happy to help you, when time allows."	"I cannot do that, but think about other solutions."	"I get results, but not in the same way as you do."

Patient Bullies

Carolyn Roark has been a nurse for more than 30 years and works in a primary care physician's office. When I told Carolyn I was including bully behavior in this book, she was eager to share several of her bully behavior experiences with me. The following are examples of patients' Brain Color bully behavior:

- A **Yellow Brainer** commented, "You don't look old enough to be doing this!"

- A **Yellow Brainer** became verbally abusive because she was upset about cost of her prescriptions.

- A **Blue Brainer** emotionally discharged all of her feelings to the nurse and the doctor, which kept them from completing their tasks at hand and communicating about the patient's health issues.

- A **Blue Brainer** became so frightened and emotionally out of control that her behavior disrupted her physical examination, upset her physician, and caused her test results to be inaccurate.

- A **Green Brainer** told the nurse as she was about to take his blood, "You only get one try!"

- A **Green Brainer** condescendingly asked the lab technician who was about to take his blood, "Are you *good enough* to take *my* blood?"

- An **Orange Brainer** was blatantly rude to the nurse and the doctor during an annual physical examination.

- An **Orange Brainer** made inappropriate and prejudiced comments about the multicultural staff members in the office.

Carolyn also said that if a patient continues to exhibit excessively inappropriate and/or rude bully behavior, the physician will document the patient's behavior, terminate the patient, and formally advise the patient about discharge from the practice with a letter sent by postal mail.

—Sheila N. Glazov

Nurse Scapegoat

by Sharon M. Weinstein, MS, CRNI, RN, FACW, FAAN

I still recall a bullying incident that occurred with one of my Blue Brain students. She was a graduate nurse in a diploma-to-baccalaureate completion program and had years of experience as an RN. She was a nurse who graduated from a 3-year diploma program—the equivalent of getting your experience in the School of Hard Knocks. She had managed patient care in a diversity of clinical settings, including emergency and critical care. Yet, as the new nurse on the unit, she was a scapegoat. The other nurses on the unit, the "Shadowed" Brain Color Bullies, decided that she was a poor fit, and they took it upon themselves to make her life miserable. The graduate nurse was diligently working to orient herself to the unit, the policies and procedures, and the culture and Brain Colors of her coworkers. She did her very best to familiarize herself with the system, and, in return, she was rewarded with stress.

My Blue Brain student was clearly bullied! She consulted with the Talent Management Department staff and determined that perhaps this job was not a good "fit" for her after all. She soon left the facility, and, in doing so, the hospital was left without a very fine, caring clinician. In this hospital, like so many others, the ratio of employees to agency staff is low. It is not a surprise that the hospital has problems retaining its own dedicated staff. It is also not a surprise that the cause of this problem is bullying.

Bully Behavior and Stress

by Sharon M. Weinstein, MS, CRNI, RN, FACW, FAAN

Causes of work-related stress include:

- Bullying.
- Being unhappy in your job.
- A heavy workload or excess responsibility.
- Working long hours.
- Poor management.
- Unclear expectations of your work.

- Lack of input in the decision-making process.
- Working under dangerous conditions.
- Insecurity about one's chance for advancement or the threat of termination.

As health care professionals, we all want to work in a positive practice environment, one with meaningful recognition for the values that we bring to the bedside or to the board room. The work environment affects patient outcomes. When we, as nurses, feel a sense of disconnect or a lack of teamwork, or perhaps that management's values are not congruent with our own, the stressors increase. Bullying increases burnout, and burnout decreases staffing—it is a vicious cycle.

To combat bullying, the institution or organization must have a "zero tolerance" mindset. Regardless of one's level within the facility, no one has the right to abuse and demean another. Both Rachel, a nurse who had relocated from a health care facility in Maryland, and Cassie, a nursing student, recognized the behavior toward them as bullying, but some nurses remain unaware that unfair or preferential scheduling, open criticism, being unapproachable, and showing favoritism to others are all forms of bullying.

And, what can the nurse do? I have found that body language can help. Yes, nonverbal behaviors communicate your message to those around you. It seems that when bullies are seeking their potential targets, they go for those who are timid, quiet, reserved, or who lack confidence. These professionals appear to be easy targets. The power stance—with chin up, eyes straight ahead, arms and shoulders in the open position, and full, determined steps—sends an important message. The power stance says, *"I am confident and not an easy target."* If the bully still approaches—stare directly at the bully and never waver. A direct stare deflects the activity, and the bully will redirect his or her efforts toward another victim.

So, the cycle begins again with another victim of the workplace bully. Dealing with disruptive behavior requires team effort on the part of staff and management—a commitment to a corporate or medical office culture that decries lateral violence and embraces fairness.

Think about spending a day in the life of a nurse—would you survive the pressure, the stress, and the bully—or would you thrive in the presence of a safe work setting?

An Angry Word

Margaret E. Bruner's poem, "An Angry Word," succinctly describes the consequences of bully behavior.

An Angry Word
An angry word is like a boomerang;
Its force returns upon the one who sent it,
And yet unlike it, for it has a fang
Whose poison doubles after one has spent it.

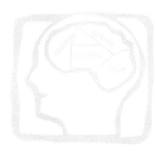

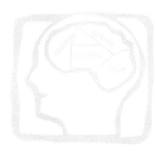

No-Brainer Conflict Resolution and Creative Problem Solving

"... if we have problems with our friends or family, we blame the other person.... Blaming has no positive effect at all ... just understanding. If you understand, and you show that you understand ... the situation will change."
—Thich Nhat Hanh, Zen Master

Unconventional Solution

by Deb Gauldin, RN, PMS

As an experienced maternity nurse with an Orange/Blue Brain Color Personality, I was practicing at a facility where women could labor, deliver, and recover in the comfort of beautifully furnished birthing suites. A lovely couple arrived on an impossibly busy evening. Women were laboring on stretchers, just waiting for suites to become available. I settled my patient into what was a makeshift exam room and noticed tears slowly rolling down her cheeks. Plans for a "natural delivery" of her first child had been derailed by a medical emergency. She described an extremely stressful and traumatic previous surgical cesarean birth and shared how much she wished for a calm, peaceful delivery with this pregnancy.

From *What Color Is Your Brain?® When Caring for Patients: An Easy Approach for Understanding Your Personality Type and Your Patient's Perspective.* Published by SLACK Incorporated. Copyright Sheila N. Glazov. http://www.sheilaglazov.com

I listened with compassion and reported to our extremely Yellow Brain and overwhelmed supervising nurse. A sterile, steel operating room was the only space available, *period*! The heartstrings of my Blue Heart nearly snapped. I simply had to draw on the spontaneous creativity that is my Orange/Blue Brain to find a better solution.

I had it! But how would I get buy-in from the rest of the team? I quickly assessed each member's Brain Color Personality and came up with a Green Brain strategy.

Convincing our Yellow Brain charge nurse to break protocol and release some control could be a challenge. She would need a detailed plan with clear steps and would want to know exactly what was expected of her. She would need reassurance that everything was under control.

The attending obstetrician was sporting a predominantly logical and traditional Green Brain, so the risk of being uncooperative about any unconventional solution was likely. To convince the doctor that *he* had come up with the solution was imperative.

The solution**:** Instead of moving the laboring woman into the cold, green-tiled operating room, I would move the necessary medical equipment into the exam room and do my best to transform the room into a smaller, yet safe, version of a birthing suite.

The Yellow Brain charge nurse saw that I had a plan that would not require her help and agreed to it, on condition that the doctor approved. I informed the Green Brain physician via telephone of his new patient, her labor status, and the census on the unit. Then I explained that an exam room was converted to a birthing room and I had secured an operating room as an emergency backup. Before he could object, I expressed concern about *his* comfort functioning in the smaller room and invited him to ask me for anything he might need to make *his* experience better. I also let him know how much the expectant couple appreciated his efforts in making this second birth experience a more positive one, even under such busy circumstances. Then I held my breath.

He thanked me for keeping him up to date on her progress and hung up. I exhaled. Next, I reassured the Yellow Brain charge nurse of his approval … and ran like the wind to actually convert the room!

One hour later, a little boy was safely delivered, tenderly swaddled, and resting in his mother's arms. Lullabies played intimately in the background as the father snapped photos. Creating a workable solution was dependent on recognizing and understanding both the "Bright" and the "Shadowed" parts of one another's behavior. This positive outcome may otherwise have been thwarted by mis-understanding and conflict.

As a side note, this happened to be the last delivery I attended before leaving the bedside to pursue a remarkably gratifying career as a singing nurse humorist. I recall welling up with tears as I sat on a stool, quietly charting in the corner of the dimly lit room. I knew my understanding of Brain Color-based behavior made a real difference to this sweet family. I felt particularly torn about my deci-sion to leave the bedside. It was just then that I heard these parents discussing the newborn's exceptionally long fingers. *"Maybe he will change the world by playing piano,"* cooed his daddy. I smiled to myself and felt the Blue part of my brain and heart melt.

Misunderstandings

Miscommunications create misunderstandings. Learning how to communicate and interpret Brain Colors will reduce conflicts and increase harmony in your life. The following no-brainer conflict resolution verse will help you remember how to avoid miscommuni-cations and misunderstandings.

> *Greens never want to be wrong and*
> *Yellows always need be right.*
> *Blues continue to talk and talk, while*
> *Oranges need to take a hike.*

The Back Story

As in a book or movie, if you get to know and understand another person's back story, you can reduce misunder-standings and miscommunications. A person's back story provides all the relevant events or circumstances that have influenced his or her point of view and behavior. Stop, think, and appreciate the fact that others may not know how or want to do things the way you would.

Misunderstandings and conflict make it difficult for individuals to appreciate their differences. The result is that they become "Shadowed" and demonstrate the fearful, negative dark side of their personality.

During my school visits and programs for adults, I introduce "Meevillain," who is the "Shadowed" character in **Princess Shayna's Invisible Visible Gift** (my children's fairy tale Brain book). Meevillain is the evil princess of the Forest of Fear. I explain that when a child or adult becomes a Meevillain, their focus is on "Me." They can be tempted to do "evil" things and become a "villain" to others and to themselves. The fun and easy-to-understand concept of "Me-evil-villain" offers the children and adults an amusing way to explain "Shadowed" and fearful behavior.

When your pediatric or adult patients and/or their family members demonstrate Meevillain's "Shadowed" behavior, their attitude about themselves and others change. They become less understanding of other people's differences. Where there had once been open acceptance and respect for others, they now have built walls of mistrust and misunderstanding.

"Wet Paint"

When our Brain Color intensifies, understanding and being compatible can be problematic. Yellow is the most intense color of the color spectrum and can be the most intense personality to work with. However, I think the following advice from my friend's mother, who was a Yellow Brainer, is remarkably wise—when you're in the midst of conflict, tell yourself or others, "I'm 'Wet Paint!' I need time to dry!"

The following is a simple explanation of "Wet Paint." When individuals are "Wet Paint," they are feeling untouchable, sticky, annoyed, and want to be left alone. They need time to slowly dry and recompose themselves. They also can give off unpleasant vibrations that cause others to stay away from them. Just like a park bench that has been painted, it needs to dry to be comfortably enjoyed, and so do individuals.

It is much easier to use the "Wet Paint" phase instead of having to explain your behavior or feelings when you do not feel like talking.

A **Yellow Brainer** may not feel like being responsible to take charge and organize a cardiac rehabilitation department holiday celebration. No explanation needed. She just needs to say, "I'm Yellow 'Wet Paint!' I need time to dry!"

A **Blue Brainer** has been up all night taking care of her sick child and comes to work not wanting to chat-chat with other nurses in the medical office. No explanation needed. She just needs to say, "I'm Blue 'Wet Paint!' I need time to dry!"

A **Green Brainer** is struggling with a new computer program that he purchased for his physical therapy office because the program has wreaked havoc with all the other programs on his computer. No explanation needed. He just needs to say, "I'm Green 'Wet Paint!' I need time to dry!"

An **Orange Brainer** is finding it difficult and feeling overwhelmed with all of the new procedures and policies in the emergency department. No explanation needed. He just needs to say, "I'm Orange 'Wet Paint!' I need time to dry!"

Compatible and Conflicting Behavior

When your Brain Color personality is feeling **Brightly Esteemed**, your behavior is positive and compatible with the other Brain Colors. However, when you are feeling like "Wet Paint," your Brain Color personality is "**Shadowed**" and your behavior is negative and in conflict with other Brain Colors. The charts on pages 190-193 show each Brain Color's **Brightly Esteemed Compatible Behavior** and **Conflicting "Wet Paint"/"Shadowed" Behavior**.

Brain Color Compatible and Conflicting Behavior

A Yellow Brainer's Compatible Brightly Esteemed Behavior	A Yellow Brainer's Conflicting "Shadowed"/"Wet Paint" Behavior
Takes care of others	Is judgmental
Is prompt	Gets sick and tired
Is loyal to family and friends	Complains "poor me"
Is organized and completes tasks	Needs to be in control
Is responsible and dependable	Is inflexible to change
Makes detailed plans	Is excessively rigid about rules
Likes to know what is expected of him or her	Worries about what will happen

Brain Color Compatible and Conflicting Behavior

A Blue Brainer's Compatible Brightly Esteemed Behavior	A Blue Brainer's Conflicting "Shadowed"/"Wet Paint" Behavior
Gets and gives hugs	Cries and may become hysterical
Cooperates with others	Repeatedly talks about problems
Enjoys life and "smells the roses"	Becomes sad and sorry
Is compassionate and truthful	Says "I am feeling OK" but is not okay
Is creative	Denies unhappy reality
Is a good listener and shares his or her feelings	Yells and screams
Trusts his or her intuition	Reacts without thinking

From *What Color Is Your Brain?® When Caring for Patients: An Easy Approach for Understanding Your Personality Type and Your Patient's Perspective.* Published by SLACK Incorporated. Copyright Sheila N. Glazov. http://www.sheilaglazov.com

Brain Color Compatible and Conflicting Behavior

A Green Brainer's Compatible Brightly Esteemed Behavior	A Green Brainer's Conflicting "Shadowed"/"Wet Paint" Behavior
Solves problems	Ignores others with a "cold shoulder"
Shows how smart he or she is	Is sarcastic and unkind
Is curious	Becomes indecisive
Is logical and precise	Does not like to make mistakes
Follows a systematic routine	Is insensitive
Likes privacy and alone time	Is uncomfortable showing emotions
Promotes fairness	Withdraws and is uncooperative

Brain Color Compatible and Conflicting Behavior

A Orange Brainer's Compatible Brightly Esteemed Behavior	An Orange Brainer's Conflicting "Shadowed"/"Wet Paint" Behavior
Demonstrates skillfulness	Acts extremely immature
Likes to have FUN!	Breaks the rules
Is courageous	Explodes with emotions
Is competitive	Does not tell the truth
Enjoys challenges	Is rude
Expresses feelings and thoughts easily	Physically acts out emotions
Acts spontaneously	Lacks self-control

From *What Color Is Your Brain? When Caring for Patients: An Easy Approach for Understanding Your Personality Type and Your Patient's Perspective*. Published by SLACK Incorporated. Copyright Sheila N. Glazov. http://www.sheilaglazov.com

Nurse's "Shadowed" Behavior

by Sharon M. Weinstein, MS, CRNI, RN, FACW, FAAN

A young nurse colleague, who recently relocated from Maryland to Illinois and applied for a staff position in a suburban hospital, shared the following story:

The young nurse was highly qualified, much more so than the nurse manager of the unit to which she would be assigned (if hired). It was clear that her Green Brain credentials presented an intimidation factor for the hiring manager, Ms. "Shadowed" Yellow Brain. Rather than offer Ms. Green Brain a position in the organization and grow from her experience, which would clearly add value to the unit and to the system, Ms. Shadowed Yellow Brain reported that the applicant was "not qualified."

Not qualified?—she was so qualified, credentialed, and experienced that she could easily have replaced Ms. Shadowed Yellow Brain as unit manager. And that, of course, was the problem. Rather than surround herself with talented professionals who could make her look good, Ms. Shadowed Yellow Brain chose to reject the applicant, and "soil" the profession.

Ask in Color

Use your Brain Colors to avoid becoming "Wet Paint" and "Shadowed." To easily resolve conflict, ask the other person to become more of another Brain Color, such as in the following examples:

- To get a job done on time, ask an **Orange Brainer** to be more Yellow and prompt.
- For more affection or compassion from a **Green Brainer**, ask him or her to be more Blue and kind.
- For some quiet time to solve a problem, ask a **Blue Brainer** to be more Green and unobtrusive.
- To complete a performance improvement project, ask a **Yellow Brainer** to be more Orange and result focused.

These examples demonstrate how to eliminate criticism and conflict and create compatibility by speaking Brain Color.

External and Internal Conflict

Different Brain Color perspectives create external and internal conflict and incompatibility, such as demonstrated in the following examples:

- A **Yellow Brainer** requires strict adherence to regulations but creates more friction with his Orange Brain staff members, who have a robust aversion to the rules.

- A **Blue Brainer** wants to discuss staff problems but creates additional tension with her Green Brain manager, who feels she should solve the problems herself.

- A **Green Brainer** remains calm during a family crisis; however, her Blue emotions tug at her heart and cause conflict with other family members.

- An **Orange Brainer's** desire to own a home health care business motivates him; however, his Yellow sense of responsibility for employees and record keeping frustrate him.

Compatible Environment

When an individual feels unworthy and lacking confidence, the problem may be that his or her Brain Color personality is feeling "Shadowed" and like "Wet Paint." This awareness can be rectified by working or living in ideal conditions, which provide an opportunity for his or her Brain Color personality to thrive and feel comfortable, bright, capable, and esteemed. Review Chapter 6: *Thrive in Ideal and Safe Conditions.* Providing a climate where individuals can feel safe and unafraid to freely explore their own ideas and feelings helps to develop their creative problem-solving techniques, improves their decision-making skills, enhances their self-esteem, and helps them to become more skillful when creatively solving problems.

Brain Color Creative Problem Solving

Brain Color Creative Problem Solving is a unique and imaginative approach to a problem or a challenge for resolving conflict that uses and values each Brain Color's perspective. This process helps people look at their conflicts from a different point of view, develop a solution, and take action to implement their innovative ideas.

The first step in Brain Color Creative Problem Solving is to identify the problem:

- **Yellow Brainers** make a list to evaluate and resolve the issues.

- **Blue Brainers** discuss the issues, evaluate the reactions of others, and make suggestions.

- **Green Brainers** identify the problem and systematically think of solutions.

- **Orange Brainers** determine a variety of resources and actions that need to be taken to resolve the problem.

The second step in Brain Color Creative Problem Solving is to discuss how to deal with the individual(s) who are causing the conflict:

- **Yellow Brainers** want to meet with the people and explain how and why their behavior is causing conflict.

- **Blue Brainers** suggest giving people the opportunity to share their feelings with a person they feel is trustworthy.

- **Green Brainers** think the people should be candidly told on a one-to-one basis about the facts and why they are part of the conflict.

- **Orange Brainers** recommend keeping an open mind, approaching the person casually, and not making a "big deal" about the conflict.

The third step after identifying the conflict and dealing with the individual(s) who cause the conflict, is to come to a consensus and/or an agreement about resolving the conflict:

- **Yellow Brainers** make sure that everyone is on the same page, following the proper procedures, and committing to the final decision.

- **Blue Brainers** want to encourage open lines of communication, exercise flexibility while listening to everyone's opinions, and maintain a cooperative attitude about the decision.

- **Green Brainers** will agree to a meeting of the minds after they have gathered all the facts, as they will remain objective and discuss the solution privately with the person who caused the conflict.

- **Orange Brainers** want to move quickly, use their master negotiating skills to resolve the problem, and keep moving on without getting stuck on past problems.

Breaking Down A Task = Success

by Kristine E. Yung, OTR/L

Sean is a 7 year old who doesn't think he will be able to ride a bike because it is too scary and he can get hurt. He is quick to respond to challenging things, such as bike riding, in a negative manner with comments such as: *"I cannot ride my bike," "I will never ever never ride a bike because I can't do it."* Sean has a wonderful sense of humor, so, by mirroring his comments with the same tone in his voice, he would laugh and realize that his statement was incorrect.

In addition, I would agree with his "can't" phrase and then repeat to him all of the other things he originally said he couldn't do but that he was doing now, such as writing, cutting with scissors, and climbing a rope wall. He would laugh and then agree to try bike riding with me.

When I broke down the steps of bike riding and told him about achieving the task in small steps, he was able to meet the challenge. So, the first time, our goal was to be able to turn the bike while walking with it. After it was achieved, he would have a sense of accomplishment, and he would be able to try the next step. Within three 45-minute sessions, he was able to ride a bike without training wheels. Breaking the task down for Sean was critical to his success due to his need to feel a sense of accomplishment of each step of the process.

A Spare Corner in Your Head

We shall always keep a spare corner in our heads
To give passing hospitality to our friends' [or other people's]
opinion.
—Joseph Joubert

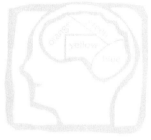

16

DECREASE STRESS AND INCREASE WELLNESS

"I'm Letting Go ..."

While traveling to Palm Springs, California, my mother was seated next to a gentleman in the first class section of the aircraft. Right after takeoff, her seatmate stretched his left arm out in front of his body and rhythmically began to open and close his fist.

My mother, who was a Yellow Brain Worrier and a Blue Brain Nurturer, became concerned and thought he was not feeling well.

"Excuse me, are you feeling okay?" she inquired.

He responded, "I'm fine, thank you. I'm just letting go of my stress and negative thoughts."

"Splendid idea," my mother replied.

Yellow Brainers find it extremely difficult not to worry because of their need to be prepared and feel in control of their lives. After that experience, whenever my mother's Yellow Brain began to worry, she would practice her seatmate's letting go technique to reduce her stress and remove troublesome thoughts.

From *What Color Is Your Brain?® When Caring for Patients:*
An Easy Approach for Understanding Your
Personality Type and Your Patient's Perspective.
Published by SLACK Incorporated.
Copyright Sheila N. Glazov. http://www.sheilaglazov.com

What a simple activity and metaphorical solution—unclench the issues you are holding on to, fan your finger apart, and free yourself of negative thoughts!

Not a Norman Rockwell Painting

Health care no longer looks like Norman Rockwell's famous 1929 painting, "Doctor and the Doll," or the family doctors of the past who lived in the same communities as their patients, made house calls, sat up all night with sick children until they passed "the crisis," delivered babies, read x-rays, splinted fractures, tended to elderly and dying patients, and soothed family members' broken hearts and spirits. The picture that was painted literally and figuratively represented the solidity and importance of comforting relationships that are embedded in a community.

Today, health care looks more like the list that follows, which could easily be a multiple choice stress test in which health care professionals check the words that relate to their workplace environment. Working in health care requires individuals to deal with some of the most stressful circumstances not found in most other workplaces. Put a check mark next to the following words or phrases that relate to the stress factors you encounter in your workplace:

- Overwork/schedule/staffing
- Performance audit
- Accreditation
- Documentation
- New technology
- Outdated equipment
- Hierarchy of authority
- Learning new skills
- Corporate mergers
- Regulation issues, either state or federal
- Demanding family members
- Patient death
- Life-threatening injuries
- Complex illnesses
- Feeling overwhelmed
- Time management issues
- Delegation of responsibilities
- Insurance companies
- Life-balance struggles
- Challenging patients

You could select any of those situations, and each Brain Color would experience that stressful workplace situation from their own perspective. You can also mix and match situations shown in the following Brain Color's Stressors chart to determine how each personality might respond to specific stressors and situations:

Brain Color Stressors

Yellow Brain	Blue Brain	Green Brain	Orange Brain
Disorganization	Poor communication	Lack of appropriate resources	Unrealistic expectations
Inaccurate directions	No cooperation	Incompetency	Arbitrary rules
No policies	Negativity	No privacy	Too many meetings
Unexpected changes	Lack of trust	Too much conversation	Lack of quick results
Tasks that waste time	"No one is listening to me!"	Mistakes	No teamwork
Incomplete records	Gossip	No time to process and solve problems	No time off or rewards
Tardiness	Selfishness	Invasion of personal space	Tedium
Others who are not prepared	Dishonesty	Giving explanations to others	Management's "red tape"
People who break the rules	Lack of compassion	Incorrect statistics or data	Inflexibility
Unreliable people and equipment	Discrimination	Repetition	Inertia

From *What Color Is Your Brain?® When Caring for Patients: An Easy Approach for Understanding Your Personality Type and Your Patient's Perspective.* Published by SLACK Incorporated. Copyright Sheila N. Glazov. http://www.sheilaglazov.com

Feeling Overwhelmed

In your health care environment, time constraints and having to perform more tasks in less time may cause individuals to feel overwhelmed. Each Brain Color has the following unique ways of dealing with feelings of being overwhelmed:

 YELLOW BRAINERS

- Make lists.
- Get organized.
- Check off their accomplishments.
- "I'll just do it myself."

 BLUE BRAINERS

- Take a break from work and then go back to tasks.
- Become exceptionally quiet.
- Talk with others about issues and ask for their perspectives.
- Sharing their emotions and concerns with a person they trust.

 GREEN BRAINERS

- Prioritize tasks logically.
- Process problem solving alone.
- Withdraw to analyze situations.
- Identify available resources.

 ORANGE BRAINERS

- Engage in a physical activity.
- "Don't worry, be happy!"
- Make time to do something fun.
- Jump in and get the job done.

Managing Your Time

Time management can be a difficult or desirable task, depending on your Brain Colors. It is vital that each Brain Color learn how to develop time management skills to decrease their stress. The following are stress-reducing examples:

 YELLOW BRAINERS

- Schedule work and play.
- Work in increments.
- Prepare tasks ahead of time.

 BLUE BRAINERS

- Just say "no."
- Enjoy a hobby.
- Plan time with family and friends.

 GREEN BRAINERS

- Their work *is* their play.
- Strategize a self-care plan.
- Schedule a time to learn something new.

 ORANGE BRAINERS

- Make "me" time.
- Spontaneously have fun.
- Design a new adventure.

Delegate and Ask for Help

If you asked yourself, "How well do I delegate responsibilities?" or "How easily do I ask for help?," you may stumble over your answers. Knowing how to delegate responsibilities and ask for help can be different and difficult experiences for each Brain Color. However, knowing why these behaviors present significant challenges for each Brain Color can reduce stress, such as described in the following examples:

- **Yellow Brainers** find it difficult to delegate responsibilities and ask for help because they want to remain in charge. To feel comfortable delegating responsibilities, they have to develop and provide others with guidelines. They have a tendency to be micromanagers because they do not think others can perform the tasks the "right way"—"my way."

- **Blue Brainers** find it difficult to delegate responsibilities and ask for help because they do not want to impose on others. They know that a coworker would help, but they feel uncomfortable asking because they know that the individual has his or her own tasks to complete, and the request might upset the coworker's schedule and cause a conflict.

- **Green Brainers** find it difficult to delegate responsibilities and ask for help because they know they are competent and do not need to ask for help. They do not want to teach a coworker how to do the job and/or deal with an individual who lacks the skills and/or knowledge to do the job as well as the Green Brainer.

- **Orange Brainers** find it difficult to delegate responsibilities and ask for help because they do not have the time or patience to deal with another individual's learning curve. They will ask a team member who they value for help and leave the job to them. Then, they are on to the next task, without checking back with their team member to make sure he or she is doing the job well.

Stress and Wellness Lessons for My Patients and Me

by Teri Elliott-Burke, PT, MHS, BCB-PMD

I own a unique physical therapy practice that specializes in treating pelvic-floor muscle disorders, including pelvic pain. Many of my patients have decreased their pain and increased their wellness by decreasing their stress. The first step in this process is the awareness of the body–mind connection of negative stress and pain; then, one can move on to fix the issue.

For example, a 49-year-old Yellow Brain executive experienced pelvic pain. The major source of the pain is tight pelvic-floor muscu-lature. Over the course of treatment, we began to notice a pattern of increased pelvic pain in this individual while she was preparing for and during a board meeting. This was especially challenging because the duration of the board meeting was a half-day and required prolonged sitting, which also increased her pelvic-floor muscle pain.

As the Yellow Brain executive became more aware of her stress–pain connection, she and I began experimenting with ways to deal with her stress. The following activities helped her to manage the situation:

1. While preparing for her meeting, she would take a break every hour and perform 5 minutes of deep breathing. She found an app called *Calm* to help her.

2. On the day of the meeting, she would rise early and walk on her treadmill for 20 minutes.

3. She talked with the person in charge of the agenda and sched-uled several breaks over the course of the meeting so she could get up and stretch.

4. After the meeting, she would schedule time with a friend or her spouse for the purpose of relaxing and laughing.

As for me, over the years of treating patients, I have noticed the stress building in my own life, often manifesting in the form of a multitude of aches and pains. Taking a page from the Yellow Brain executive's experience, I have developed my own Green Brain stress management system:

1. At the beginning of my day and again at lunch, I practice 5 min-utes of deep breathing, which significantly relaxes my nervous system.

2. I changed my diet by decreasing sugars and increasing vegetables.

3. I perform strength training two times per week.

4. I took a more active approach to my schedule, limiting the num-ber of patients I see in one day and taking extra time for lunch a couple of days per week.

5. I reflect on the positive impact that my care has had on others.

6. I spend time with family and friends who make me laugh.

7. Speaking of laughing, I bought Bill Cosby's old routines on CD [compact disc], and when I need a good laugh, I listen to those. Not only are they funny, but they also remind me of my childhood when my family would listen to Bill and crack up!

The preceding Green Brain system is not perfect for the times I still find myself overwhelmed. But overall, I rarely take a sick day, I have lost a few pounds on purpose, and I feel good. I "snap" less at my dear husband at the end of my day and have more positive interactions with my staff. I have enjoyed the changes in my life as a result of stress management, and I hope to keep up those routines.

Use the following spaces and your Green Brain to develop your own system to decrease stress and increase wellness in your life:

1. _____
2. _____
3. _____
4. _____
5. _____

Keep Your Energy Up and Your Stress Down

Not delegating responsibilities and asking for help are just two behaviors that can increase your stress and decrease your energy. Recognizing and knowing how you and the other Brain Color personalities respond to stressful situations regarding wellness and safety will help you to keep your energy up and your stress down. This information will also help you to understand how to reduce stress, increase your energy and comfort to help you create a positive perspective about your patients' and their family members' attitude about wellness.

Keep Your Energy Up and Your Stress Down

Yellow Brainers	Blue Brainers	Green Brainers	Orange Brainers
Finishing projects on time	Helping others	Reading	Exercising
Completing tasks without errors	Talking with patients and coworkers	Learning about new technology	Making exceptions to the rules
Streamlining procedures	Using creativity to solve problems	Utilizing innovative technology	Making workspace the way *they* want it
Encouraging safety in the workplace	Relaxation breaks (e.g., yoga, workouts)	Scheduling quiet time	Exploring new opportunities
Striving for financial security	Listening to music	Researching data to solve problems	Enjoying the unexpected
Cleaning his or her workspace	Personalizing his or her workspace	Accomplishing tasks efficiently	Requesting flexible work time
Reorganizing his or her workspace	Creating colorful workspace or uniform	Problem solving with logic and facts	Having social time with coworkers
Being prepared	Preparing healthy homemade meals	Staying within a budget	Changing work schedules or responsibilities frequently

From *What Color Is Your Brain?® When Caring for Patients: An Easy Approach for Understanding Your Personality Type and Your Patient's Perspective.* Published by SLACK Incorporated. Copyright Sheila N. Glazov. http://www.sheilaglazov.com

Making A "Healthy Decision"

We all find it difficult to sometimes say "no" to other people's requests. Many years ago, my Blue Brain learned to say, "Thank you for asking. However, your request is not a healthy decision for me." Sometimes my answer bewilders people and they ask me what it means; other times, they are so surprised that they just stop asking. During these times, I have a serious conversation with myself to decide whether what I am in a quandary about is a "healthy" decision for me. I consider these queries to be self-caring not self-centered.

I also share this healthy way of saying no and the decision-making tip with my clients and program participants. At first, some people hesitate to use the new phrase. However, after a few attempts, they tell me that they find it easier to say no and are happier because they are taking good care of themselves physically, emotionally, financially, and/or spiritually.

Taking Good Care of Yourself

Taking good care of yourself is easier for some Brain Colors than for others. It is beneficial to learn how each personality masters the art of being self-caring and apply that information to your life.

Yellow Brainers often have to force themselves to be self-caring. They esteem themselves by being responsible and never want to appear unreliable. They take good care of themselves by preparing a schedule to exercise, making healthy meals, and organizing their home.

Blue Brainers may struggle with learning to be self-caring. They esteem themselves by being compassionate and never want to appear as selfish. They take good care of themselves by doing something they enjoy, such as yoga, walking outside with a friend or pet, and/or spending time with loved ones.

Green Brainers logically know they should take care of themselves. They esteem themselves by being independent, but they can become focused on their work and do not bother to take care of themselves. They take good care of themselves by reading, spending time by themselves, and researching new ways to exercise and eat well.

Orange Brainers like their "me" time to take care of themselves. They esteem themselves by being resourceful and finding ways to stay healthy so they can continue to be active and have fun. They take good care of themselves by going on vacations, enjoying athletic activities, and not "sweating the small stuff."

A Journey to Wellness

by Virginia Schoenfeld, PhD, BCC

Wellness means different things to different people, including health care professionals. Wellness is not just the absence of disease, but it is a commitment to making necessary lifestyles changes. I am a wellness coach, and in my practice I encourage clients to think of wellness as a fluid process, one that is multidimensional (mind, body, spirit), where the client is accountable and responsible for the outcomes.

The path is challenging for clients. One of my clients—I will call her "Jane"—came to see me for stress reduction. A friend had told her about our B.R.E.A.T.H. Wellness Center, which offers integrative health services at a low or no cost to military and low income individuals. Jane had served in the military as a medic but was discharged for medical reasons; the VA [Veterans' Administration] had later determined that she had anxiety disorder, PTSD [posttraumatic stress disorder], depression, and suicidal ideation.

Jane was also given multiple prescription medications to control her symptoms, which included inability to sleep, overconsumption of alcohol, lack of motivation, and low self-esteem. When I first met with her, I asked why she thought I could help her.

She did not know what to expect from wellness coaching sessions, but she realized that "coaching" did not carry with it the dark cloud that mental health counseling did. Jane learned that wellness was multidimensional and that at some point we would have to address her eating habits; she would have to learn how food is connected to brain performance and proper functioning of all body systems.

During the intake, she mentioned that she had allergies and knee pain, but she did not want to focus on them, just on her emotional wellness. After Jane identified her goals for our sessions, her VA physician and I began to collaborate to support our client. Jane wanted to find meaning in her life, get a job, and get off medications. She was taking 15 different psychotropic medications when we first started. However, 1 year and several coaching sessions later, Jane's physician gradually lowered the dosages and discontinued some of her medications.

Today, at her request, Jane is down to three medications and very low dosages. Her sleep improved, she went back to school, got her own residence, and started a new job just in the past 3 months! We went from weekly sessions to monthly sessions. Things were going great ... at least that is what I thought until 2 weeks ago when I received a telephone call late on a Friday afternoon from Jane. She sounded flustered and had been crying. She wanted to see me when she was finished work. I accommodated her the same day because I did not know what to expect. She had never cried in any of her sessions, but she was crying now.

Being in the military and growing up in a family that said, "kids do not cry," Jane found crying to be a weakness, and her personality had always come across as extraordinarily tough. When we met, I knew there had been a huge release of energy, starting at the core of who she was.

During our session, Jane said, 'My new job sucked, my allergies got worse on the job, I could not relate socially to my coworkers, and I reported to a much younger supervisor. It was not for me, so I quit!'

During our "crisis" session, we reviewed Jane's initial wellness goals, and I asked her if she needed to update them. I could see that Jane was moving toward a different understanding of wellness! Jane had ignored the importance of food in her wellness journey, but she was now ready to make the changes needed to reclaim her health. Jane returned to my office 1 week later with two completed assignments—a 5-day food journal and a self-evaluation of her career and social needs, using Maslow's hierachy of needs model.

As a coach, I knew the "energy" had shifted when Jane declared, "While doing my food journal, I realized for the first time that I could not find healthy foods in my kitchen or refrigerator."

Jane was so concerned with this fact that she ran to the grocery store to buy vegetables and fruits. For the first time, we laughed together about her discovery. My heart was convinced that Jane was finally on her way to a higher level of wellness. She had learned many de-stressing tools during the past year, which improved her sleep, motivation, and outlook in life, but now she was seeing the whole picture clearly.

Jane understood the need for creating healthy habits, attempting new things, accepting life's challenges, and practicing self-love. Jane also learned that her healing journey is about connecting mind, body, and spirit, thus achieving allostasis [maintaining stability through change]. Jane is not finished with her wellness journey, but she is on her way!

How Do You Live Your Life?

"How you start your day is how you live your day,
And how you live your day is how you live your life."
—Louise L. Hay, author of *Heal Your Body A-Z*

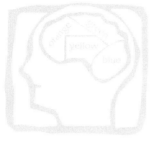

17

You Can Change Your Brain Color

"We cannot change anything until we accept it. Condemnation does not liberate, it oppresses."
—Carl Jung

Hospice Nurse and Daughter

by Anonymous Hospice Nurse

Half of my nursing career has been spent as a hospice nurse. My role has been as a Blue Brain coach to families and patients facing life-limiting illnesses, working with them to meet the goals and challenges they face as they attempt to embrace the impermanence of life and the struggle to let go.

Working with people from all walks of life and embracing their differences, values, and goals is where I have found my Blue Brain passion. This role often requires that I change my temperament, thus transforming me to flow with the changes that patients and their families are experiencing. This transformation, which varies from home to home, can be demanding, but at the same time it has allowed me to have some of the most glorious interactions with people. I have spent time sitting on the floor next to the rocking chair of a 92-year-old man listening to stories of Omaha Beach, listening to stories from an elderly Dutch woman of how as a child

From *What Color Is Your Brain?® When Caring for Patients: An Easy Approach for Understanding Your Personality Type and Your Patient's Perspective.* Published by SLACK Incorporated. Copyright Sheila N. Glazov. http://www.sheilaglazov.com

she ran from rooftop to rooftop when German solders knocked on the door of her home during World War II, and listening about the hopes and dreams of a 20-year-old young man who will never know the fulfillment of his dream of becoming a jazz pianist but still sharing the dream in his words and images. Not all encounters are calm and reflective. I have been challenged in many homes, such as when walking into a home of a family in which siblings are at odds and the resultant sense of bitterness that engulfs me when I cross the threshold.

At a time when so many things are out of control, patients and families look to me to provide moments of guidance and instruction, allowing them to take back some of the control they have lost. These challenges and the changes faced by others have contributed to the work in progress that I am. I have come away from each and every interaction with a new piece of myself, and I have been privileged to share in these many lives for an instant in time.

The moment came to use what I had embraced in my vocation and face one of the greatest changes in my life. My father had suffered for years due to the effects of diabetes and eventual renal failure. At the age of 69, after 13 years of dialysis, he chose hospice care, exercising what little control he had to choose death *on his terms.* We spent the final 2 weeks of his life on earth together as a family. My parents' home was a revolving door of friends and family saying their good-byes and sharing the final moments of his life. When he finally took his last breath, there were feelings of immense pain, as well as relief—relief that his suffering had ended and pain from the loss of his physical presence. Losing my father was one of the most difficult experiences and abrupt changes in my life. The weeks I spent with my father and being present at the time of his death was one of the greatest gifts he gave to me. This gift ultimately helped me to meet the challenge of the changes I would face—embracing the impermanence of life, letting go of the physical, and keeping with me the essence of his life.

Reviewing Change

The following is a review and a reminder of previous chapters that discussed how individuals from each of the Brain Colors handle change from their own perspective:

- **Yellow Brainers** must *plan* for change. To be comfortable, they need to feel that they are in control of the change.
- **Blue Brainers** must *feel* good about a change. To be comfortable, they need to trust their intuition about the change.
- **Green Brainers** must *think* about change. To be comfortable, they need to gather and contemplate all the facts before they consider making a change.
- **Orange Brainers** *are* the change agents. To be comfortable, they constantly need to create change. They cannot stand boredom.

Life Changes

Lifelong experiences and maturity offer us new opportunities to modify our Brain Colors and/or change them to the opposite Brain Color, such as described in the following:

- **Yellow Brainers** can become more Orange. They no longer have to be as responsible to their family, careers, or community as they did when they were younger. With their children grown, they feel it is their time to have new adventures. They have the resources to take some risks and the time to have more fun.
- **Blue Brainers** can become more Green. They no longer have to nurture others. They can be self-caring and focus on themselves. They take good care of themselves by going back to school, focusing on a new career, or delving into a hobby that earlier required too much time or money.
- **Green Brainers** can become more Blue. They no longer have to be focused on solving business or family problems. They have amassed a lifetime of knowledge and experience, but they no longer need to impart it to others. They have opportunities to show the sensitive Blue facet of their personality.
- **Orange Brainers** can become more Yellow. They actually become tired of taking risks and want more security. They are comfortable not being the "crazy one" in their family or circle

of friends. Although they still like to march to a different drum, they modify their brisk tempo to a slower pace.

Environmental Changes

An environment can influence how you can change your Brain Color. As I entered the lobby of my client's office building, my Yellow Brain began to shift to Blue. A colorful decor and pictorial history of the company greeted me as I walked toward a large cafeteria, which faced a landscaped garden adjacent to my destination. The meeting room contained a gallery of employees with smiling faces.

The color scheme was teal and cranberry, accented by soft lighting. Upholstered chairs surrounded the tables, which allowed the attendees to make eye contact during the program. The comfortable and calming environment enhanced the attendees' attention and ability to learn about the following environments in which individuals can comfortably change their Brain Colors:

 YELLOW BRAINERS CAN CHANGE IN A:

- *Yellow*, well-organized situation.
- *Blue* situation that encourages a traditional, family-type atmosphere.
- *Green* situation that maintains a systematic routine.
- *Orange* situation that has a "game plan."

 BLUE BRAINERS CAN CHANGE IN A:

- *Blue* environment that is friendly.
- *Yellow* environment that has day care for their children.
- *Green* environment that appreciates their authenticity.
- *Orange* environment that acknowledges their social contributions to the group.

 GREEN BRAINERS CAN CHANGE IN A:

- *Green* setting that is efficient.
- *Yellow* setting that values consistent quality.

- *Blue* setting with smart people.
- *Orange* "virtual" setting that requires no meetings.

 ORANGE BRAINERS CAN CHANGE IN A:

- *Orange* atmosphere that is stimulating and high-spirited.
- *Yellow* atmosphere that provides an opportunity for physical activity.
- *Green* atmosphere that values direct responses.
- *Blue* atmosphere that encourages imagination.

Shifting Your Point of View

To adapt to change, individuals often have to shift their point of view (POV) to feel comfortable with and adapt to the adjustments they foresee and/or will have to make.

Yellow Brainers can shift their POV if they feel they have some influence over the change.

Blue Brainers can shift their POV if their emotional concerns about the change are validated.

Green Brainers can shift their POV if they have been given substantial facts for the change.

Orange Brainers can shift their POV if they know their sense of autonomy will not be limited.

Stress and Change

Dealing with change and the stress it creates can be an exciting challenge or a dreadful curse, depending on each Brain Color's perspective.

Yellow Brainers are anti-change at almost any cost. When they do have to change, they deal with the stress of change by developing procedures to feel secure and responsible about the change process.

Blue Brainers enjoy change because they think of change as a creative process. They deal with the stress of change by harmoniously meeting others' halfway and thinking about how they would feel if they were in another person's situation because of the change.

Green Brainers like change and the innovative opportunities that it offers. They deal with the stress of change by retreating into their own quiet place of comfort, without any distractions, to think about the effects the change will have on them.

Orange Brainers welcome change and are the change agents. They deal with the stress of change by using it as a vehicle to reach their goals, challenging themselves, and/or turning the changes into a competition to determine how fast they can adapt.

Leadership and Change

If you are in a leadership role or in a situation that determines you are the person who must introduce change to your team, the following tips will help you to handle the responsibility. It is important for you to remember that these Brain Color introductions also are examples of how each Brain Color likes to learn about and process their ideas about change.

Yellow Leaders introduce and like to learn about change with detailed explanations about the who, what, why, when, and where of the change.

Blue Leaders introduce and like to learn about change by sharing ideas with their team, letting team members voice their concerns, and giving the team reassurance that, as their Blue Leader, they will be available for assistance.

Green Leaders introduce and like to learn about change by precise statements of facts, the purpose, and the proposed outcomes of the change.

Orange Leaders introduce and like to learn about change, with explanations of the "What's in it for me and my colleagues" point of view, and challenges of the change.

Responding to Change

by Denise Knoblauch, BSN, RN, COHN-S/CM

Medical offices, clinics, and hospitals are rapidly changing from paper charting to the electronic medical record. Ideally, the charts will link to a patient's records and involves an integrated health care system for patient care. This process often seems extremely rigid and inflexible because patients have to fill in the blanks and complete all the questions, even if the questions are not pertinent to them. For example, an outpatient may have to adapt and answer questions related to inpatient care for safety and compliance for hospital accreditation or Medicare and/or insurance purposes. Many patients find it difficult to respond to this change. They become aggravated because of the duplication of questions. This change also requires medical staff to spend extra time at the computer inputting information and making sure the documentation is correct, which can make a patient think that the health care provider is not paying attention to or about his or her issues.

Each Brain Color's response to change demonstrates their attitude and acceptance of the change process and how it affects them.

Yellow Brainers respond to change by being adaptable if they feel safe and secure about the change.

Blue Brainers respond to change with sensitivity about how the change affects themselves and others.

Green Brainers respond well to change if it solves a problem and makes sense.

Orange Brainers respond quickly to change and embrace the new opportunities.

A Growing Challenge

Whenever a life experience or having to change my Blue Brain Color has challenged me, I encourage myself with one of my favorite affirmations:

"It was gruesome and I grew some.
In fact, I should be 10 feet tall by now."

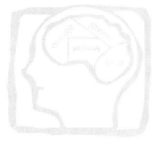

18

EFFECTIVE DECISION MAKING AND MOTIVATION

*"It's not hard to make decisions
when you know what your values are."*
—Roy E. Disney

Knowing your Brain Colors makes it easier to recognize your values and make decisions. Every day we confront issues and make decisions that are stressful and can affect our health.

Diabetes has become a worldwide health care epidemic. According to the World Health Organization, 347 million people worldwide have diabetes, and it is expected to affect 552 million by 2030 (http://www.who.int/mediacentre/factsheets/fs312/en/). Stress has a tremendous effect on blood sugar levels and diabetes management. The following vignettes demonstrate how relationships can create stress, especially when the individuals are not aware of each other's Brain Colors and what they value.

Blue and Green Brain Decisions and Stress

A wife thinks she is being thoughtful when she asks her husband how his blood sugar levels have been. He tells her, "Second-guessing my diabetes management is unnecessary; you should know I'm not stupid. I can take care of myself!"

221

"You don't appreciate me," she sobs. "It takes time to shop, pre-pare, and cook all the appropriate foods for you, and you don't even notice!"

The husband ignores his wife and retreats to his garage workshop to tinker with his motorcycle. If the wife knew her husband was a **Green Brainer**, she would have understood his need for privacy and sense of competency about his diabetes management. If the husband knew his wife was a **Blue Brainer**, he would have recognized that she asked him about his diabetes because she wanted to be helpful and demonstrate her love and concern for his well-being.

Their Brain Color knowledge would have reinforced the hus-band's and wife's appreciation for each other's values and attitude and shown them how they each could contribute to the husband's optimal diabetes management.

Yellow and Orange Decisions and Stress

A father thinks he is doing the right thing when he tells his teen-age daughter who has Type 1 diabetes, "I know what is best for you; you *must* keep a detailed record of your meals, exercise, and glucose levels in your online log book."

His daughter wails, "I'm furious with *you*, *your* rules, and *your* intrusion in *my* life." Then she stomps off to her bedroom, slams the door, and calls her best friend to complain about her father "who treats me like a baby!"

If the father knew his daughter was an **Orange Brainer**, it would have reinforced the fact that **Orange Brain** teenagers are highly impulsive and loathe parental lectures. If the daughter recognized that her father was a **Yellow Brainer**, she would know he needed to be a **Yellow Brain** responsible parent and coach her about a game plan to responsibly manage her diabetes. Their Brain Color knowl-edge would have helped the father and daughter to be receptive to each other's values and attitudes about living a healthier life.

Live a Healthier Life

by Carole Childers, LDN, CN

It is no secret that we all make countless decisions every day—from the monumental and life changing, to the simple and mundane. In fact, we can't live without making decisions. Everything we do, say, or think involves a decision. Yes; even breathing is a decision.

Making decisions is stressful and can stifle our motivation to act or follow through with our choices. Constantly dealing with this stress weakens our immune system. We become vulnerable to all sorts of medical problems, which, of course, create even more decisions for us to make under even more stressful conditions.

The health connection to motivating ourselves to healthier decisions lies in reducing the stress associated with our choices. Managing our stress in reasonable ways improves our health. When we are healthier, we feel better, stronger, wiser, have more energy, and are more motivated and productive. Consequently, we are able to make better decisions and follow through with them in our everyday lives, both personally and professionally. We even become more persuasive as positive role models for our patients.

Managing Stress When Making Decisions

Can we simply just decide to make stress go away? Wave a magic wand and Poof!—stress-free living permanently appears? It doesn't quite work that way. But there are some things we all can decide to do to enhance the quality of the decisions we make and to help each of us make more of the right decisions that will improve our personal lives and our professional performance.

It begins with one very important, yet often relegated or sometimes neglected, decision—*deciding to live a healthier life*! It is not about the latest fad diet or exercise craze. It is about taking a kind and loving look at ourselves and our lifestyle. Go to the mirror and ask:

Do I look healthy?

- Is my skin clear and vibrant?
- Do I have dark circles under my eyes?
- Am I overweight? Is my hair shiny?

Do I feel healthy?

- Am I tired all the time?
- Do I lack energy?
- Do I feel irritable or over stressed?

Am I healthy?

- Do I know my blood sugar level?
- Do I know my cholesterol levels?
- Do I have high blood pressure?
- Can I climb the stairs without breathing hard?
- Do I have any food or chemical sensitivities?

Answering these questions should give you a fair idea of how the decisions you are making are affecting your health. Deciding to live healthier will motivate you to make better decisions that ultimately improve your health and quality of life. Living a healthier life will help you to be stronger, have more energy, think more clearly, and handle the stress of making those hard choices when they come your way. You will also be creating a positive role model for your patients.

Motivation for Making Healthier Decisions

There are three basic components of your lifestyle that you can change for the better: sleep, nutrition, and exercise. The following are some helpful tips for all three:

Sleep: Getting Enough of It

Your body needs 7 to 8 hours of deep, refreshing sleep every night. Lack of sleep can lead to overeating and affect the quality of decision making. Lack of sleep also affects the way you look and feel. You are tired, lack energy, and are irritable.

What to do: Disconnect Yourself

- Set a time to turn off all cell phones, tablets, computers, televisions, and radios at least 30 minutes before bedtime.
- Be aware of how caffeine affects you and when you consume it.
- Do not exercise just before bedtime.
- Stop eating at least 1 hour before bedtime.
- Indulge in a relaxing tub bath before going to sleep.
- Learn to perform meditation and deep breathing exercises, even in the middle of the day.

Nutrition: Our Society is Addicted to Processed Foods, Fat, and Sugar

We often eat for comfort and stress relief.

What to do: Small Changes Make Big Differences

• Need to lose weight? Don't go on a crash diet. Losing one or two pounds per week is weight you will not gain back.

• Eat a complete protein (e.g., eggs, chicken, turkey, beef, fish, and beans and rice in combination) three times per day to sustain your energy.

• *Your mom was right.* Breakfast *is* the most important meal of the day. Quality protein shakes are a quick and easy way to start your day.

• Evaluate what and when you're eating, your quality of nutrition, portion sizes, and how often you snack.

• Drink enough water. Drink half of your body weight in ounces of water every day (e.g., 140-pound adult = 70 ounces of water). Coffee, tea, and soda do NOT count.

• Get off diet soda. Aspartame breaks down chemically into formaldehyde. *Why would you want to pickle your brain before you are done using it?*

• Avoid eating on-the-run or out of a vending machine. Plan healthy meals ahead of time. Chicken for dinner tonight? Cook an extra chicken breast for tomorrow's lunch.

• If you work in an office where "reps" often bring in lunch, ask them to cut back on the carbohydrates and increase the protein.

• Find a quiet place to eat lunch, away from the stress of your desk. Stress negatively affects digestion.

• Start Office Salad Days. Have everyone in the office bring an ingredient. Dressings always on the side for dipping, never on the salad.

Exercise: Get up and MOVE

We are a nation of couch potatoes who are addicted to the latest in high-tech entertainment. We constantly eat, sleep, and think with electronic laborsaving gadgets. Exercise is good for you; not only can it help you lose or maintain your proper weight, but it can help you to increase your energy, boost your mood, improve your sex life, and generally help you to prevent or manage a wide range of health problems.

What to do: Make a Plan and Get an Exercise Buddy

- It is important that you are active regularly. Aim for at least 20 to 30 minutes of activity every day.

- The best time to exercise is on an empty stomach, such as first thing in the morning before eating breakfast or in the evening before eating dinner.

- Exercising with a friend or a group of friends will help you to stay motivated as you support each other and enjoy sharing the fun.

- Be flexible. If you cannot find time for your regular workout, improvise—take the stairs instead of the elevator, park at the far end of the lot, or amp up the pace of your household chores.

- Remember, any physical activity is much better than no activity at all.

- Join a health club, a YMCA, a dance class, or a local activity club, such as Masters Swimming or a USA Cycling club. Group activities keep you motivated and inspire new social connections.

- Remember to check with your health care professional before starting any new exercise program, especially if you have not exercised for a long time or have chronic health problems.

Needless to say, deciding to live healthier takes work, but we all can agree that reducing stress is a better way to live a longer, happier, and successful life. I hope these tips will motivate you to start. If you need more help, contact a nutritionist in your area. Remember, modeling a healthy lifestyle creates a mirror for motivating your patients to make better decisions on reaching their own goals.

Whatever your Brain Color, put it to good use to motivate yourself to achieve the healthy lifestyle that suits you best and the one you deserve!

The **Brain Color Effective Decision Making** chart on page 227 will help you to reflect on your decision-making process during stressful or tranquil situations.

Brain Color Effective Decision Making			
Yellow Brainers	**Blue Brainers**	**Green Brainers**	**Orange Brainers**
Create a detailed plan	Use their hearts, not their heads	Researches facts	Stay in the moment
Thinks through all ideas	Tells others about ideas	Analyze statistics	Improvise when necessary
Execute in a timely manner	Wants other people's opinions	Apply formulas	Look at competition
Do not procrastinate	Go with intuitive feelings	Project outcomes	Ignore fear
Say, "We must go by the book."	Say, "Consider the consequences to others."	Say, "Let's look at and evaluate the finances."	Say, "If you've got the money, use it!"
Deliberate outcomes	Do not consider costs an issue	Create systems	Pay no attention to consequences

From *What Color Is Your Brain?® When Caring for Patients: An Easy Approach for Understanding Your Personality Type and Your Patient's Perspective.* Published by SLACK Incorporated. Copyright Sheila N. Glazov. http://www.sheilaglazov.com

Motivate Your Brain

If you are motivated to shift your Brain Color, you can successfully change your behavior, effectively make decisions, resolve conflicts, and reduce the stress in your life. To motivate yourself or others, you need to understand the appropriate Brain Color motivators.

 YELLOW BRAINER MOTIVATORS

- Doing what is right
- Completing a to-do list
- Deadlines
- Respect
- Symbolic recognition

 BLUE BRAINER MOTIVATORS

- Others listening to and valuing my ideas
- Opportunities to share my feelings
- Not being taken for granted
- A pat on the back
- Creative opportunities

 GREEN BRAINER MOTIVATORS

- Problem-solving opportunities
- Creating a system or procedure
- Feedback at the end of a project
- Cutting-edge resources
- Recognition of my solution

 ORANGE BRAINER MOTIVATORS

- Thrill of a new challenge
- Financial rewards
- Rapid results
- Competition

Motivation in the Workplace

It is valuable to know what motivates you to make effective decisions. It is critical to understand what you can do to stay motivated and eager to do your best in your health care workplace.

Yellow Brainers stay motivated by:

- Keeping a positive attitude.
- Scheduling time off to recharge.
- Taking on a task; "I know I can do it!"

Blue Brainers stay motivated by:

- Performing tasks they enjoy doing.
- Developing friendships with other team members.
- Tapping into their creativity.

Green Brainers stay motivated by:

- Taking continuing education classes.
- Being able to research new ideas.
- Scheduling time to read books and articles.

Orange Brainers stay motivated by:

- Doing something new every day.
- Scheduling daily fun and/or exercise.
- Enjoying social activities with team members outside of work.

Motivating Others

It is beneficial to know what motivates you, and it is essential to understand what you can do to encourage your coworkers and team members to be motivated and enthusiastic about their health care responsibilities.

Yellow Brainers encourage their team members by:

- Praising and acknowledging their achievements.
- Demonstrating excellent workplace behavior.
- Expecting the best from their team members.

Blue Brainers encourage their team members by:

- Making and/or giving "good job" gifts.
- Sharing inspirational stories and poems.
- Being interested in their family and life outside of the workplace.

Green Brainers encourage their team members by:

- Setting reasonable goals that team members can meet and be successful.
- Offering incentives and educational opportunities.
- Providing fair feedback.

Orange Brainers encourage their team members by:

- Scheduling team celebrations.
- Having contests within the department.
- Giving camaraderie pep talks.

Motivating Quiet Hands With Hula Hoops

by Kristine E. Yung, OTR/L

Personal space is a challenging concept for some children to learn and difficult for other children to recognize. My favorite story about personal space involves a couple of boys who would walk down the hall of my clinic with their hands dragging on the wall. It was as if the wall or their bodies would fall over if their hands were not on the wall.

We talked about "quiet hands," which is a silly term that we use for those who have the ability to not touch other people or objects. So, it became my challenge to help the boys understand the concept of personal space. I gave each of the boys a hula hoop and asked them to sit inside of it. After they were inside, we talked about it being our "space house" and that the walls were fragile, like a bubble. When another person comes into our house, the walls will break, just like a bubble pops. We practiced moving around the room, avoiding touching one another to keep our bubbles safe. After we completed the "outer space walk," pretending that we are exploring the moon, we sat down.

I explained that something had happened to our personal space bubbles and we all needed to get into the small hula hoop. The boys were excited over the new twist in the play, and they climbed into the hoop. But the excitement of the potential doom soon filled them with the complaints of "Evan is touching me," "Ashton is stepping on my foot," and "Ms. Kris, can I get out of here, I can't breathe?"

The small space bubble had served its purpose—to teach them about how it feels to have personal space invaded. The two boys I originally practiced this game with did not walk with their hands touching the wall from that point forward. A simple reminder about the space bubbles and the hula hoop was the only cue that was needed to help them with their body position.

Confusion and Clarity

Confusion can be a powerful motivator and can influence our decision-making process, and if we are willing to be uncomfortable and patient, we can make a "healthy decision" for ourselves.

Many years ago, my Green Brain friend, Gordon Alper, offered me long-lasting advice: "*Sit with confusion like a brick in your lap.*"

My Blue Brain modified Gordon's advice. Now our combined advice is: "*Sit with confusion like a brick in your lap.* **Out of confusion comes clarity.**"

After you have clarity, it is much easier to make a Healthy Decision. Often, people respond to a question or request without considering whether their response is a "healthy decision" emotionally, physically, spiritually, or financially.

Remember, after you have clarity, it is much easier to be motivated and make effective and "healthy" decisions.

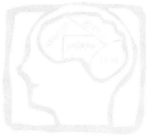

CLUES, QUOTES, AND FAMOUS PERSONALITIES

A Green/Blue Brainer confided in me, saying, "I went through life doing and saying things but not knowing why. I'm no longer color blind; the Brain Colors cured me and gave me the answers too!"

With the following collection of Brain Color quotes and clues, you will be able to recognize other Brain Colors when you meet or interact with them in your health care workplace, at home, or in your community. Just for fun, I have included a list of Brain Color quotes, clues, and distinguished health care professionals, including nurses, physicians, researchers, and famous people and their careers, according to my **WCIYB?** research and the concepts.

Yellow Brainer Quotes, Clues, and Famous Personalities

Yellow Brainer Quotes

- "The baby was born at the wrong time; it messed up my schedule during the big selling season."
- "I come in a half hour before work to stock towels, fill our receipt book with totals, and enter them into the computer."

- "I can't stand the money not facing up; it all should be facing the same way!"
- "Yellow people are 'T' crossers and 'I' dotters."
- "I'm Rependable! That means I'm responsible, respectful, accountable, and dependable." (I promised Eric, a fifth grader, I would always give him credit when I used his word.)
- "I organize, supervise, delegate, follow up, and reinforce."

Yellow Brainer Clues

- They forward "neatnik tips" to friends and family.
- They are worriers. *You* do not have to worry; they are worrying for you.
- They often seem rushed; their need to stay on schedule and complete everything on their to-do list is a priority.
- They find it hard to control their urge to straighten pictures on a restaurant wall, lamp shades in the hotel lobby, or decorative pillows on a friend's living room sofa.

Distinguished Yellow Brain Health Care Professionals

Nurses

- Mary Breckinridge (1881-1965), founder of the new model of rural health care and the Frontier Nursing Service
- Mary Eliza Mahoney (1845-1926), first African American Registered Nurse
- Hazel W. Johnson-Brown (1927-2011), first African American Chief of the Army Nurse Corps
- Anna Caroline Maxwell (1851-1929), founder of the Army Nurse Corps

Physicians and Researchers

- Dr. John Morgan (1735-1789), founder of the College of Philadelphia Medical School (now the University of Pennsylvania School of Medicine), which was the first and only medical school in the original 13 American colonies

- Dr. Alois Alzheimer (1864-1915), first to record his descriptions and discoveries and diagnose a disease of the brain that was later named after him
- Dr. Nathan Smith Davis (1817-1904), founder of the American Medical Association

Famous Yellow Brainers
- President George Washington (1732-1799)
- General Colin Powell (1937-Present)
- Prime Minister Margaret Thatcher (1925-2013)
- Emily Post (1872-1960), etiquette expert
- Samuel Moore Walton (1918-1992), founder of Wal-Mart

Blue Brainer Quotes, Clues, and Famous Personalities

Blue Brainer Quotes
- "I love you more than tongue can tell!"
- "Every year when new interns arrive, we give them the Brain Color quiz and explain how we use it in the agency."
- "I need a real person! I don't want to talk to a tech person or go to a website."
- "My friends are the people who know the songs in my heart and sing them to me when I forget the words."
- "It's easy to speak my mind, because it comes straight from my heart."

Blue Brainer Clues
- They leave "love notes" in their loved ones' lunch bags, suitcases, kitchen cabinets, or briefcases.
- They want peace at any price; however, they usually pay a huge price.

- They can drive themselves, as well as others, crazy (especially the Green Brainers) when they reiterate their issue of concern or idea repeatedly while trying to solve a problem.

- They expect people to be honest and are disappointed when they are not.

Distinguished Blue Brain Health Care Professionals

Nurses

- Dorothea Dix (1802-1887), passionate teacher and advocate for the first mental asylum in the United States

- Margaret Sanger (1879-1966), founder of Planned Parenthood

- Susie King Taylor (1848-1912), first African American U.S. Army Nurse in the U.S. Civil War

- Helen Fairchild (1885-1918), frontline combat nurse in World War I

Physicians and Researchers

- Dr. Elizabeth Blackwell (1821-1910), first female doctor in America. Blackwell viewed medicine as a means for social and moral reform and believed that women would succeed in medicine because of their humane female values. Emily Blackwell, Elizabeth (Emily's sister), and their colleague, Marie Zakrzewska, founded the New York Infirmary for Women and Children, the first American hospital run by women and the first dedicated to serving women and children.

- Dr. Mary Putnam Jacobi (1842-1906), physician, author, scientist, researcher, activist, medical educator, and pioneer focused on curing disease. She believed women should participate as the equals of men in all medical specialties and was married to Dr. Abraham Jacobi, founder of the discipline of pediatrics.

- Dr. James Blundell (1791-1878), physician, physiologist, obstetrician, teacher, innovator, and pioneer who was the first physician to successfully achieve a blood transfusion on one of his obstetric patients.

Famous Blue Brainers

- President Abraham Lincoln (1809-1865)
- Mother Teresa (1910-1997)
- Martin Luther King, Jr. (1929-1968)
- First Lady Eleanor Roosevelt (1884-1972)
- Robert Frost (1874-1963), poet

Green Brainer Quotes, Clues, and Famous Personalities

Green Brainer Quotes

- "I'm glad my kids are smart, because I would not have tolerated it if they were dumb."
- "I wish everyone would stop bothering me; I value my alone time."
- "I am going to do something ***ungreen*** and give you a hug."
- "I need to know that...why? And it affects me...how?"
- "Anytime I can solve a problem, it's a good day!"
- "I don't need to know what doesn't pertain to me; the less I know about others, the better."

Green Brainer Clues

- They do not have to like or have a relationship with others to work with them.
- They want to get all the facts from other people, but they don't give the facts to others: "We don't want them to know what we know, but we want to know what they know."
- They are proficient at remembering data—dates, numbers, years, places, and facts. They are big winners at the game *Trivial Pursuit*.
- They like people to come to them with questions, but they can be condescending with their answers.

Distinguished Green Brain Health Care Professionals

Nurses

- Florence Nightingale (1820-1910), founder of modern nursing
- Mabel Keaton Staupers (1890-1989), strategically led the battle to end racial prejudice in nursing and built a secure platform for African American nurses
- Virginia Avenel Henderson (1897-1996), known as First Lady of Nursing and developed a nursing theory known as the Henderson model
- Elizabeth Grace Neill (1846-1926), developed the system of nursing registration

Physicians and Researchers

- Sir Frederick Banting (1891-1941), physician, painter, and Nobel laureate. He and Dr. Charles Best, a medical student who was his assistant, isolated the internal secretions of the pancreas and discovered insulin.
- Marie (1867-1943) and Pierre (1859-1906) Curie, Nobel Prize winning physicists and chemists, who researched and experimented with radioactive substances and invented the word "radioactivity." Pierre worked with Marie to isolate and discover radium and polonium.
- Dr. Louis B. Newman (1900-1992), mechanical engineer and physician who skillfully combined knowledge and experience to become a pioneer and one of the founding fathers of physical medicine and therapy.

Famous Green Brainers

- President Thomas Jefferson (1743-1826)
- Frank Lloyd Wright (1867-1959), American architect
- Dr. Jonas Salk (1914-1995)
- Bill Gates (1955-Present)
- Thomas Edison (1847-1931)

Orange Brainer Quotes, Clues, and Famous Personalities

Orange Brainer Quotes

- "I can pretty much do anything, so you can carry on and I will be brilliant!"
- "I put pending projects in subdivided piles that are moved to the corner of my office. It's the only space in my office. Visitors can't see the piles, but I can!"
- "My life has been crazy and my Orange Brain is probably overcommitted."
- "I don't have to explain my behavior—they have to explain theirs."
- "I've worked in the unpredictable emergency department for 23 years!"

Orange Brainer Clues

- They look at life as a verb, not a noun.
- They do not want details; just give them the bottom line.
- They think if they obey all the rules, they will miss all the fun.
- They do not want to be paralyzed by policies.

Distinguished Orange Brain Health Care Professionals

Nurses

- Clara Barton (1821-1912), founder of American Red Cross
- Sarah Emma Edmonds (1841-1898), a clever Union nurse who disguised herself as a man to infiltrate the Confederate lines during the U.S. Civil War
- Colonel Ruby Bradley (1907-2002), Army Nurse Corps. Most decorated woman in U.S. military history, receiving 34 medals and citations of bravery for her military service during World War II and the Korean War and was known as an "Angel in

Fatigues" during her imprisonment in the Japanese Santo Tomas Internment Camp in Manila, Philippines. Her awards included Legion of Merit Medals, Bronze Stars, Presidential Emblems, the WWII Victory Medal, the U.N. Service Medal, and the Florence Nightingale Medal.

- Diane Carlson Evans (1946-Present), Vietnam War nurse and Founder and President of Vietnam Women's Memorial Foundation

Physicians and Researchers

- Sir Joseph Lister (1828-1912), surgeon and pioneer of antiseptic surgery. He applied Louis Pasteur's (chemist and microbiologist) advances in microbiology to promote his theories of sterile surgery. He is known as the "Father of Asepsis."

- Earle Dickinson (1892-1961), invented the Band-Aid brand of adhesive bandages, or plasters, while employed by Johnson & Johnson. When his wife found it difficult to use gauze and bandage dressings after cutting her fingers, Earle attached some gauze to adhesive tape and kept it sterile by adding crinoline.

- Dr. Edward Jenner (1749-1823), physician who conducted an experiment on one of his patients to prevent him from dying from smallpox. He inoculated the boy with cowpox when he became ill and then inoculated him with smallpox, creating the world's first vaccine. The boy survived and Dr. Jenner became known as the Father of Immunology.

Famous Orange Brainers

- President Bill Clinton (1946-Present)
- Lee Iacocca (1924-Present), American businessman
- Prime Minister Golda Meir (1898-1978)
- Amelia Earhart (1897-1939), American aviation pioneer
- John Glenn (1921-Present), astronaut

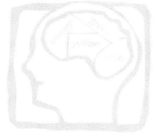

INSIDE MY SHIRT
IS .....

My Blue Brain perspective views a celebration as a beginning, not an ending. Yes, this is the ending of the book. However, it is the beginning of your "Happy Brainday" celebration, where you are the guest of honor. Congratulations!

You have learned the fundamental Brain Color concepts when caring for patients and learned how to understand and value yourself and others, resolve conflicts quickly, build harmonious relationships, and improve your health care job performance. I encourage you to continue honoring yourself and celebrating your Yellow, Blue, Green, and Orange Brain Strengths and Perspectives. They are color-filled "Praiseworthy Gifts" you can share with others and use in your professional and personal life.

Have fun being who you are! Think about your Brainday as a birthday, which, by definition, is a day commemorating the founding, or beginning, of something. Unlike a traditional once-a-year birthday, you can celebrate a Happy Brainday every day!

I feel blessed to have an abundance of Brainday and birthday memories. One of my favorite memories is of the sixth birthday party of our youngest son, Noah. Noah celebrated his birthday as the ringmaster of 12 other 6-year-old guests who brought him a battalion of GI Joe figures, a squadron of superheroes, and loads of Legos.

The last gift was a shirt with an iron-on appliqué that read: "**Inside This Shirt Is One Terrific Kid!**" His eyes sparkled like the candles on his Superman cake as he examined his gift—stretching the neckline, peeking inside each armhole, and tugging open the bottom of the shirt. However, his smile quickly became a frown.

"Noah, why such a sad face?" I asked.

"Mommy, where's the kid?" Noah asked, offering me his shirt.

I realized that Noah literally thought a new pal was hiding inside his shirt. Of course, it made perfect sense to an Orange/Blue 6 year old! However, I knew that putting on his new shirt would erase his frustration. He wriggled into his shirt with his head and arms popping out like a little painted turtle. Then he posed as his favorite superhero, a mini-Superman, patting his chest with pride and exclaiming, "It's me!"

When I tell this story at the conclusion of my **WCIYB?** Programs, I never fail to hear "ohs" and "awws." I use a replica of Noah's favorite childhood article of clothing because he wore his "It's me!" shirt until it became too small and threadbare.

However, I have changed the wording to: **Inside My Shirt Is One Terrific Kid!** Then I conclude the program with an invitation to the attendees to think about their own "Praiseworthy Gifts" and give themselves an "It's me!" gift and fill in the blanks in their workbook or handout.

When I remind people to think about their own "Praiseworthy Gifts," some individuals are perplexed or feel awkward. Most individuals can tell you what is remarkable about their loved ones, friends, or colleagues, but they usually never think about what is remarkable about themselves, as they would consider it to be too self-centered. I believe it is self-caring to acknowledge your own remarkable Brain Color attributes and abilities and "Praiseworthy Gifts."

I invite you to think about your "Praiseworthy Gifts" in your health care workplace. You might like to change "terrific" to another adjective that describes you more appropriately. You might prefer the terms *creative, smart, organized, exciting, responsible, flexible, funny, competent,* or *courageous.* You also might be more comfortable changing "kid" to person, nurse, physician, doctor, therapist, health care team member, medical office staff member, technician, medical assistant, physician's assistant, or any of the many health care professions titles.

Write the words that work best for you and your Brain Colors:

Inside My Shirt Is One _____ _____!

As you begin your day and are deciding what to wear to begin you day, shift your Orange Brain into high gear— become a kid and have some fun. Transform yourself into a superhero! Imagine wearing a Yellow, Blue, Green, or Orange Brain Color t-shirt underneath your clothing or wear some article of clothing or accessary that complements your Brain Color. You will begin the day knowing that you gave yourself an *"It's me!"* gift.

SECTION III: BRAIN COLOR COMMUNICATION AND COLLABORATION SUMMARY

Brain Color Communication	Yellow Brainers	Blue Brainers	Green Brainers	Orange Brainers
Ask About Other People's	Home and community	Family, friends, and pets	Education and favorite books	Hobbies and vacations
Listen, They Say...	"Should"	"Love"	"Think"	"Fun"
Telephone Good-Byes	"Be careful"	"I love you" or "take care"	Don't say anything; they just hang up	"Enjoy"
Communication Clues	Be polite Stay on track Tell them details	Use stories Connect personally	No "small talk" Be brief Give statistics	Be direct Quick to the point Give results
Tone of Voice	Diplomatic	Cooperative	Informative	Encouraging
Approach With Others	Formal	Friendly	Academic	Relaxed
Understand Their...	Commitment	Sensitivity	Brevity	Spontaneity
Mottos	"Follow the rules."	"We can help each other."	"Think it through, thoroughly."	"Let's go for it!"

(*continued*)

From *What Color Is Your Brain?® When Caring for Patients: An Easy Approach for Understanding Your Personality Type and Your Patient's Perspective*. Published by SLACK Incorporated. Copyright Sheila N. Glazov. http://www.sheilaglazov.com

SECTION III: BRAIN COLOR COMMUNICATION AND COLLABORATION SUMMARY (continued)

Brain Color Communication	Yellow Brainers	Blue Brainers	Green Brainers	Orange Brainers
Excellent Patient Care	Understand they are upset about not feeling in control	Let them talk about their concerns for family and pets	Explain medical strategies to solve health problems	Acknowledge their frustration about being confined
Make Patient Feel Comfortable	Make sure the patient feels safe	Ask the patient how he or she is feeling	Let the patient know you are capable	Respond to the patient's needs as quickly as possible
Improve Patient Satisfaction	Hold staff accountable	Share test results	Identify barriers	Encourage staff by offering rewards
Stressors	Tasks that waste time	Lack of compassion	Invasion of personal space	Arbitrary rules and restrictions
When Feeling Overwhelmed	Make lists	Let go of emotions	Withdraw to analyze the situation	"Don't worry, be happy!"
Manage Time	Work in increments	Learn to say "no"	Strategize self-care plan	Make "me" time

(continued)

From *What Color Is Your Brain?® When Caring for Patients: An Easy Approach for Understanding Your Personality Type and Your Patient's Perspective.* Published by SLACK Incorporated. Copyright Sheila N. Glazov. http://www.sheilaglazov.com

SECTION III: BRAIN COLOR COMMUNICATION AND COLLABORATION SUMMARY (continued)

Brain Color Communication	Yellow Brainers	Blue Brainers	Green Brainers	Orange Brainers
Keep Energy Up and Stress Down	Streamline procedures	Personalize workspace	Stay within the budget	Flexible work time
Bully Behavior	Demonstrate they are in control	Make others feel badly or guilty	Intimidate others with a sense of superior intelligence	Physically dominate others
How to Deal With Negative Behavior	Understand they do not have all the details you have	Do not take their actions personally	Ignore the bully	Let negativity roll off their backs
Brightly Esteemed Compatible Behavior	Takes care of others Is prompt Knows expectations	Good listener Shares feelings Trusts intuition	Is curious Follows routine Promotes fairness	Is skillful Enjoys competition Is courageous
"Shadowed" or "Wet Paint" Behavior	Judgmental Inflexible Complains	Sad and sorry Pretends they're "OK" Denies reality	Is sarcastic Withdraws Ignores others	Breaks rules Emotions explode Is rude

From *What Color Is Your Brain?® When Caring for Patients: An Easy Approach for Understanding Your Personality Type and Your Patient's Perspective.* Published by SLACK Incorporated. Copyright Sheila N. Glazov. http://www.sheilaglazov.com

(continued)

SECTION III: BRAIN COLOR COMMUNICATION AND COLLABORATION SUMMARY (continued)

Brain Color Communication	Yellow Brainers	Blue Brainers	Green Brainers	Orange Brainers
Creative Problem Solving	Make lists to evaluate the issues	Evaluate others' reactions	Identify problems systematically	Determine resources and actions
Decision Making	Execute in timely manner	Consider how it affects others	Consider projects outcomes	Ignore fear
Motivation	Symbolic recognition	Creative opportunities	Recognition of solutions	Rapid results
Change	Plan for it	Feel good about it	Think about it	Do it
Change and Stress	Needs to feel secure	Consider how others feel	Retreat without distractions	Use change as a vehicle to reach goals
Clues and Quotes	"Yellow people are 'T' crossers and 'I' dotters." "It messed up my schedule."	"I love you more than tongue can tell." "I need to talk to a real person."	"I wish everyone would stop bothering me." "I'm glad my kids are smart."	"I can pretty much do anything!" "I am not being belligerent."

(continued)

From *What Color Is Your Brain?® When Caring for Patients: An Easy Approach for Understanding Your Personality Type and Your Patient's Perspective.* Published by SLACK Incorporated. Copyright Sheila N. Glazov. http://www.sheilaglazov.com

SECTION III: BRAIN COLOR COMMUNICATION AND COLLABORATION SUMMARY (continued)

Brain Color Communication	Yellow Brainers	Blue Brainers	Green Brainers	Orange Brainers
Famous Nurses	Mary Breckinridge Mary Eliza Mahoney Hazel Johnson-Brown	Dorothea Dix Margaret Sanger Susie King Taylor	Florence Nightingale Mabel Keaton Staupers Elizabeth Grace Neill	Clara Barton Sarah Emma Edmonds Diane Carlson Evans
Famous Physicians and Researchers	John Morgan Alois Alzheimer Nathan S. Davis	Elizabeth Blackwell Mary Putnam Jacobi James Blundell	Fredrick Banting Marie & Pierre Curie Louis B. Newman	Joseph Lister Earle Dickinson Edward Jenner
Famous People	George Washington Colin Powell Sam Walton	Abraham Lincoln Mother Theresa Martin Luther King, Jr.	Thomas Jefferson Thomas Edison Bill Gates	Bill Clinton Amelia Earhart Lee Iacocca
Inside My Shirt Is One...	Organized department manager	Compassionate physical therapist	Competent diabetes educator	Funny pediatric nurse

From *What Color Is Your Brain?® When Caring for Patients: An Easy Approach for Understanding Your Personality Type and Your Patient's Perspective.* Published by SLACK Incorporated. Copyright Sheila N. Glazov. http://www.sheilaglazov.com

Bibliography

Brizendine, L. (2006). *The female brain.* New York: Morgan Road Books.

Carter, R. (1999). *Mapping the mind.* Berkeley: University of California Press.

Keirsey, D., & Bates, M. (1984). *Please understand me: Character and temperament types.* Del Mar, CA: Prometheus Nemesis.

Lindsey, J. S., & White, K. R. (2015). *Take charge of your healthcare management career: 50 lessons that drive success.* Health Administration Press.

Moire, A., & Jessel, D. (1992). *Brain sex: The real difference between men and women.* New York: Dell Publishing.

Tannen, D. (2001). *You just don't understand: Women and men in conversation.* New York: HarperCollins.

The Joint Commission. (2007). *What did the doctor say?: Improving health literacy to protect patient safety.* Oakbrook Terrace, IL: The Joint Commission. Retrieved from http://www.jointcommission.org/assets/1/18/improving_health_literacy.pdf

OTHER BOOKS, CDS, AND DVDS YOU MIGHT ENJOY

Bell, A. H., & Smith, D. M. (2004). *Difficult people at work: How to cope, how to win.* New York: MJF Books.

Brinkman, R., & Kirschner, R. (2003). *Dealing with difficult people : 24 lessons for bringing out the best in everyone.* New York: McGraw Hill.

Campbell, J., & Cousineau, P. (1990). *The hero's journey: Joseph Campbell on his life and work.* New York: Harper & Row.

Balnicke J., & Kennard D (directors). (1988). *Joseph Campbell: The hero's journey* [documentary]. United States: Acadia.

Campbell, J., & Moyers, B. (1991). *The power of myth.* New York: Doubleday.

Chiazzari, S. (1998). *The complete book of color: Using color for lifestyle, health, and well-being.* Boston: Element.

Conroy, E. (1921). *The symbolism of color.* London: Rider.

Foster, D. G., & Marshall, M. (1994). *How can I get through to you? Breakthrough communication beyond gender, beyond therapy, beyond deception.* New York: Hyperion.

Ginott, H. G. (1969). *Between parent and child.* New York: Avon Books.

Goodman, E., & O'Brien, P. (2001). *I know just what you mean: The power of friendship in women's lives.* Parsippany, NJ: Fireside.

Isay, J. (2007). *Walking on eggshells: Navigating the delicate relationship between adult children and parents.* New York: Flying Dolphin Press.

Jung, C. G. (1964). *Man and his symbols.* New York: Doubleday.

Keirsey, D. (1998). *Please understand me II: Temperament, character, intelligence.* Del Mar, CA: Prometheus Nemesis.

Legato M. J. (2005). *Why men never remember and women never forget.* Emmaus, PA: Rodale.

Miller, M. *Brainstyles: Change your life without changing who you are.* New York: Simon & Schuster.

Moyers, B., Campbell, J., & Lucas, G. (1988). *Joseph Campbell and the power of myth* [documentary]. United States: Mystic Fire Video.

Myers Briggs, I. (1995). *Gifts differing: Understanding Personality type.* Mountain View, CA: Davies-Black Publishing.

Nierenberg, G. I., & Calero, H. H. (2004). *How to read a person like a book.* New York: Barnes & Noble.

Pease, A., & Pease, B. (2001). *Why men don't listen and women can't read maps: How we're different and what to do about it.* New York: Broadway.

Ritberger, C. (2000). *What color is your personality.* Hay House, Inc.

Rossbach, S., & Yun, L. (1997). *Living color: Master Lin Yun's guide to Feng Shui and the art of color.* New York: Kodansha America.

Zichy, S. *Women and the Leadership Q: Revealing the Four Paths to Influence and Power.* New York: McGraw-Hill.

Index

An Interview With the Author

How did the idea for the original *What Color Is Your Brain?*® (WCIYB?) book and *What Color Is Your Brain?*® *When Caring for Patients: An Easy Approach for Understanding Your Personality Type and Your Patient's Perspective* come about?

The natural progression of my **WCIYB?** Programs and people asking me for information about **WCIYB?** generated the idea to write the original book. The idea to write *What Color Is Your Brain?*® *When Caring for Patients: An Easy Approach for Understanding Your Personality Type and Your Patient's Perspective* was initiated by John Bond, Chief Content Officer/Senior Vice President at SLACK Incorporated. SLACK delivers the best in health care information and education worldwide. I have many health care clients, and writing this new health care focused book, after the success of the original book, was a "no-brainer."

I believe writing a book is like falling in love—it happens when you are ready. The right time to write the words for both books arrived and I was ready!

Initially, the original **WCIYB?** was an introductory mini-program for my strategic planning/creative problem-solving programs. Because of my education, teaching experience, and professional development courses, I knew I could offer my clients another creative problem-solving technique that was easy and uncomplicated for adults and children to learn.

Program participants enjoyed learning about the Brain Colors, and soon clients requested longer professional and personal development programs. The more programs I facilitated, the more people asked for a **WCIYB?** book.

The first edition of ***Princess Shayna's Invisible Visible Gift*** was published in 1997, and the second edition was published in 2012. The book is the fairy tale adaptation of **WCIYB?** for children of all ages. Working with the children, their parents, and their teachers offered me more opportunities to facilitate programs and presentations. The customized **WCIYB?** workbooks, all the data I compiled observing people's actions, listening to their conversations, and capturing ideas in a journal, on cocktail napkins, dining receipts, and scraps of paper became the research material I used to write **WCIYB?**

Besides a focus toward the health care audience, what make this book different from the original WCIYB?

What makes this book so different and dynamic are the 27 health care professionals, who generously contributed their authentically written anecdotal stories. Their vignettes provide powerful professional lessons that readers can relate to and will be inspired by!

How have your previous professions prepared you for your current career?

My parents and husband exemplified and encouraged my tenacity, creativity, and adventurous entrepreneurial spirit, which prepared me for my previous professions and career as an author.

I loved teaching elementary school, high school English as a Second Language, and creativity classes at several colleges and universities. I had studied psychology and various personality type indicators and learned to recognize and understand different personality types and adapt to their learning styles in a variety of environments.

I was a student of customer safety and service when my husband and I owned and operated an aviation business (commuter airline, air ambulance, flight training, air charter and rental, ground and maintenance services) and managed the county airport in Mammoth Lakes, California.

As a professional speaker, I have been privileged to work with a diverse group of clients (health care, educator, banks, association, students, corporations, parents, and veterans) in the United States, Canada, Europe, and South America. My clients taught me about their fields of expertise, the students enriched my life while I was in their classrooms, and I enjoyed teaching them how **WCIYB?** could improve their lives.

Each career change in my life, has offered me opportunities to interact with and study each Brain Color, which has enhanced my professional and personal life and craft as a writer.

Which career would you say had the most influence on you?

Each of my careers has provided me an abundance of lessons. However, I have always thought of myself as an educator. I feel my teaching experiences and relationships with my clients and students have influenced me the most.

I am a passionate educator who loves gardening inside and outside the classroom. I enjoy planting seeds of knowledge, even though I may or may not have the joy of nurturing a seedling, watching it grow, and seeing the beauty of its blossom. However, I have had the pleasure of meeting former students and maintaining relationships with clients. It is encouraging and joyful to learn how our experiences together have influenced their lives and mine.

This was true when I recognized one of my former students. He was a participant in a professional development program many years after he was a student in a third grade class I had taught. My Blue heart sang when he realized who I was and said, "I acquired my love for learning in your third grade classroom." In addition, a thank you note from a fifth grade Green Brain student is one I will cherish forever, and it sits in a beautiful frame on my desk. The message is what teaching is all about... "You are an author who brightens my path, who let me think, who made me strong, and who let me be the way I am. Thank you, Max."

From your perspective as a teacher, how do you think WCIYB? can help children learn to get along better with their peers, parents, and teachers?

WCIYB? teaches children the new three R's: Responsibility, Respect, and Relationships. During a school visit, a sixth grader once told me, "When you know your Brain Colors, you learn how to be responsible for the changes in your life and how to respect people who are different than you...be nice to other people, even when there are obstacles in your life."

Children and parents get along better with each other because they understand one another's Brain Colors and know how to speak BCSL—Brain Color as a Second Language. Recently, a friend shared his "Aha" moment with me: "For years I was perplexed because my child acted so differently from the rest of our family. Now, it all makes sense. I get it…he's Green."

WCIYB? also helps children to become responsible risk takers versus children at risk. They develop a healthy level of self-esteem, which makes them feel capable, worthy, in control, and empowered at school, at home, and in their communities. Most children create their self-image from what others (friends, parents, teachers, family members) say about them or how they react to their behavior. When students discover their Brain Colors, they also recognize their significant individual "Praiseworthy Gifts," meaningful attributes, and abilities for themselves. Their discoveries and decisions are their own and are not influenced by their teachers, parents, friends, or other family members.

Several years ago, a reading specialist wrote about the impact that **WCIYB?** had on her students. She said, "The self-esteem lessons the children have learned are like peeling back the layers of an onion and enjoying the many layers. They really feel good about themselves and the real-life skills they learned. The students speak from their hearts and their faces light up."

What are your favorite parts of sharing the WCIYB? concept with different audiences?

I love sharing **WCIYB?** with different audiences and knowing they have achieved their goals. Three of my favorite reasons for working with adult audiences are:

- Enjoying the contagious laughter that fills a room after people discover their Brain Colors. They start comparing Brain Colors with the people around them. It's fun to hear: "No wonder we get along so well, we're exactly the same!"

- Listening to program participants begin to analyze their family members and friends, such as, "I married a **Yellow Brainer** and have three Orange Brain children."

- Observing how quickly participants transfer their Brain Colors from the workplace to their home. "I have to be Green at work, but I get to be Blue at home!"

When working with children, four of my favorite times have been:

- Watching the students come to class wearing a specific Brain Color tee shirt. "We're having a math test today, so I wore my Green Brainer shirt."

- Helping the children make a Brain Color/Princess Shayna patchwork quilt. I was surprised and honored when the class presented their quilt to me as a gift.

- Sharing Brain Color/Princess Shayna Celebrations with the students, their teachers, and their parents. In one classroom, we all enjoyed yellow pineapple pieces, blue berries, green grapes, and orange slices while the children entertained us with their hilarious family Brain Color stories.

- Working face-to-face with Mrs. Laura Newcomer's enrichment classes, as well as working with Mrs. Leigh Cassell's second grade class, the teachers, and the students at Stephen Central Public School, Crediton, Ontario, Canada, via Field Trip Zoom video conferencing. We created remarkable Kingdoms of Kindness for all the students, along with wonderful hands-on learning activities and Brain Color projects. A testament to the impact of *Princess Shayna's Invisible Visible Gift* and the Brain Colors is a message I received from a Green Brain 5th grade boy in Mrs. Newcomer's class, who wrote, "You are an author who brightened by path, who let me be me, who made me strong, and who let me be the way I am. Thank you!"

How can WCIYB? help people to achieve harmony in their home, between siblings, or between spouses?

To achieve harmony at home, I encourage adults and children to remember that **WCIYB?** is an explanation, not an excuse for poor behavior. The following are two examples: "I'm not intruding on your Green privacy, I'm just being Blue" and "I'm Orange, so I don't have to follow your Yellow rules."

Family conflict is often the result of a common misconception. Adults and children think "They are my family and they should automatically understand my behavior." Consequently, a "soul mate" can become a "cell mate," and "my buddy" can become "the bully." Recognizing the different Brain Colors can help family members resolve conflicts quickly and easily. Adults and children do not blame one another because they learn to understand the other person's perspective, strengths, values, needs, priorities, stress factors, and frustrations.

It takes time and effort to recognize, acknowledge, and appreciate other people's Brain Color attributes and abilities. However, when you do, you create a cooperative and comforting home environment with your siblings and spouse.

How can WCIYB? help people to improve their health care workplace environment?

If people utilize their Brain Colors to reduce stress, create ideal and safe workplace conditions, and establish effective teamwork, they can improve their health care workplace environment and the care they offer to their patients.

Reducing stress by modifying workplace dynamics and diffusing problematic situations is easier when individuals know why they are compatible and incompatible with specific coworkers, patients, managers, and agency representatives. The Brain Colors help them to distinguish who are the "doubters" versus the "doers" and the "talkers" versus the "thinkers."

WCIYB? can be utilized as an assessment for efficient job evaluation, staffing, working with patients and their families, and create ideal working conditions in which each Brain Color thrives. For example:

- Health care leaders and managers are **Yellow Brainers** who require job description manuals.
- Health care social workers are **Blue Brainers** who need genuine feedback.
- Medical technicians are **Green Brainers** who like systems and data.

- Emergency Medical Technicians and Emergency Department staff are **Orange Brainers** who excel in obtaining immediate results.

To build a successful Brain Color team in a hospital, medical office, or health care facility, it is beneficial to establish effective teams in a collaborative environment. Understanding how to connect with and motivate each team member is significant for success.

- A **Yellow Brainer** will be on time for meetings and help organize a plan.
- A **Blue Brainer** will encourage brainstorming and communicate ideas.
- A **Green Brainer** will develop an efficient strategy to execute the plan.
- An **Orange Brainer** will enthusiastically promote ideas and get the results needed to be successful.

Implementing the **WCIYB?** concepts will increase productivity, save time and money, improve patient care, and create a collaborative health care workplace environment.

Why are you allocating a percentage of the royalties from the sale of all of your books to the Juvenile Diabetes Research Foundation (JDRF)?

I allocate 10% of the royalties to JDRF because of my commitment to help find a cure and offer comfort, education, and encouragement to children and their families who live with the never-ending challenges of diabetes.

I am not a researcher who works to find a cure for diabetes; however, I am a writer who writes the words that create a greater awareness about diabetes, and the sale of those words provides financial support to help find a cure.

I also want to honor and acknowledge our elder son, Joshua, who was diagnosed with T1D (Type I diabetes) when he was 15 years old, my father who had T2D (Type 2 diabetes), and the millions of children, adults, and their families worldwide who deal with the daily "highs" and "lows" of diabetes.

About the Author

Sheila N. Glazov is an award-winning and internationally known author, personality type expert, professional speaker, and passionate educator. Sheila's programs and books help individuals to increase harmony, collaboration, and effective communications and decrease misunderstandings and conflicts in their workplaces, homes, schools, and communities.

Sheila has appeared on CNN, NBC, ABC, FOX, LIFETIME, and WGN TV. She has been interviewed on radio stations nationwide and has been featured in the Wall Street Journal, the Chicago Tribune, the Chicago Sun Times, and the Daily Herald newspapers, Selling Power, American Society of Training and Development, HR, Women's World, Seventeen, and Enterprising Women magazines, as well as the Discover Card and Quill Corporation national customer newsletters. Today's Chicago Woman newspaper selected Sheila as one of "100 Women Making A Difference."

Sheila's innovative style has won her praise for her **What Color Is Your Brain?**® programs in conference rooms and classrooms in the United States and around the world. Encouraging adults and children to recognize and respect the best in themselves and others is the essence of her programs and books.

Sheila's programs offer practical, easy to remember, and immediately applicable concepts from her best-selling book, *What Color Is Your Brain?® A Fun and Fascinating Approach to Understanding Yourself and Others*. Throughout Sheila's programs, individuals learn to utilize their own "Instant Personality Decoder," to recognize and value their personal perspective, accept and appreciate others' viewpoints, and build healthier and more productive relationships in their professional and personal lives. Sheila offers customized **What Color Is Your Brain?**® professional development, leadership, teamwork, sales, teacher, student, parent, author, romance, family, women veterans, and women's retreat programs.

What Color Is Your Brain?® has been translated and published in Portuguese and Chinese.

Sheila's book, ***Princess Shayna's Invisible Visible Gift*** is the children's version of **What Color Is Your Brain?**®. This enduring and enlightening "family fairy tale" helps children of all ages to recognize their Brain Color capabilities, value their worthiness, build their self-esteem, develop creative problem-solving skills, and appreciate diversity. Sheila believes that every child deserves to feel loved, safe, encouraged, and confident within a trustworthy home, school, and community environment.

The ***Teacher's Activity Guide for Princess Shayna's Invisible Visible Gift*** is the perfect, quick, and easy resource to apply, transfer, and reinforce the Invisible Visible Gift valuable lessons in your classroom. Complete with Gift Giver's Guide bonus questions, Brain Color quizzes, coloring and work sheets, word games, puzzles, recipes, and 70+ time tested activities!

Princess Shayna's Invisible Visible Gift has also been adapted into two engaging and educational children's musical performances for schools and family audiences. The productions present meaningful messages about acceptance and appreciation of diversity and bully prevention.

Purr-fect Pals: A Kid, A Cat & Diabetes is engaging story told through the experiences of a Kid and a Cat, who learn to live with the everyday, challenging "highs and lows" of their Type 1 diabetes. The characters' mirror images and the sequence of events teach children that they are not alone. Readers realize they can achieve their heart's desire and overcome obstacles, turning them into life-long opportunities.

Sheila earned her Bachelor of Science degree in education from the Ohio State University, a degree in Creative Leadership from Disney University, and is a graduate of the Creative Problem Solving Institute and the McNellis Creative Planning Institute. She has taught the third grade and high school English as a Second Language. Sheila has been an adjunct faculty member of William Rainey Harper College and a guest instructor at DePaul, Penn State, and Northwood Universities.

Sheila and her husband, Jordan, live in the Chicagoland area.

To learn more about Sheila, her books, and programs visit her websites: http://www.sheilaglazov.com and http://www.Princess-Shayna.com.

Other Books Written by Sheila N. Glazov

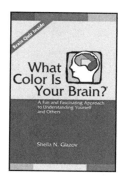

What Color Is Your Brain?® A Fun and Fascinating Approach to Understanding Yourself and Others. This book explores the essential pieces of the puzzle that is human interaction. With the help of this dynamic book, discovering your own Brain Color and learning to adapt to others is bound to be a no-brainer! The short chapters are easy to read and chockfull of intriguing facts and helpful tips that make people's complex personalities less confusing and simple to understand. Readers discover their Brain Colors and learn communication skills, just like multiplication tables, which they will never forget!

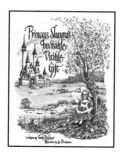

Princess Shayna's Invisible Visible Gift. This children's chapter book version of **What Color Is Your Brain?**® is not a predictable fairy tale about a princess who is saved by a prince. The enduring heroine's loving parents teach her to be a strong, independent, and self-confident young woman, whom girls and boys alike can emulate and respect. The book's lifelong lessons help children to achieve a greater understanding of themselves and others, reduce bully behavior, accept and appreciate diversity, deal with life's challenges, and celebrate life's triumphs.

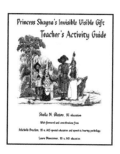

Teacher's Activity Guide for "Princess Shayna's Invisible Visible Gift." The perfect well-researched and time-tested companion for **Princess Shayna**. This quick and easy resource helps teachers and parents to apply, transfer, and reinforce meaningful messages in the classroom. Complete with Gift Giver's Guide Bonus

Questions, Brain Color quizzes, coloring and work sheets, word games, puzzles, recipes, and 70+ time tested activities!

Sheila allocates 10% of the royalties from the sale of **What Color Is Your Brain?**®, Princess Shayna's Invisible Visible Gift, and the Teacher's Activity Guide to the Juvenile Diabetes Research Foundation

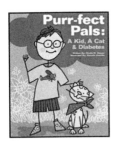

Purr-fect Pals: A Kid, A Cat & Diabetes. This unique picture, activity, and resource book was designed to offer comfort, education, and encouragement to children and their families who are newly diagnosed or have been living with the everyday challenges of Type 1 diabetes (T1D)and Type 2 diabetes (T2D). The story is told through the true-life experiences of a Kid and a Cat, who learn to live with the "highs and lows" of diabetes and teach children that they are not alone.

Sheila allocates 100% of the royalties from the sale of ***Purr-fect Pals: A Kid, A Cat & Diabetes*** to the Juvenile Diabetes Research Foundation.

For information about purchasing Sheila's books, visit http:www.sheilaglazov.com/booksdvd

What Color Is Your Brain?® Programs for Heath Care Professional Development

Sheila N. Glazov makes the art of understanding yourself and others fascinating and fun. You and your fellow health care professionals will immediately benefit from Sheila's innovative and participatory programs, which are always interactive and engaging but never tedious or tiresome. Sheila personalizes every program to satisfy each health care client's unique culture, environment, meeting, or conference.

The content of Sheila's programs is relevant, achieves constructive, long-term outcomes, and promotes enthusiastic participation. Participants quickly transfer and apply their new Brain Color knowledge to their health care workplace. Sheila can adapt her programs to provide attendees with continuing education units.

What Color Is Your Brain?® Program participants will:

1. Assess their "Health Care Professional" personality and determine their Brain Color attributes and abilities
2. Increase their awareness and appreciation for coworkers' differences and opinions
3. Create caring, collaborative, and harmonious relationships within their health care facility
4. Understand each Brain Color communication style to meet other people's needs
5. Build rapport and appropriately approach patients to offer exceptional care
6. Recognize and appreciate their "Praiseworthy Gifts"
7. Eliminate stress and solve problems by understanding patients' and coworkers' personalities and perspectives

This [Brain Color] information will be used for communicating with all the different personality types. Knowing how a person sees and feels about things helps you know how to approach the person with whom you may have issue. You may also use this information to get 'buy-in' on a

particular idea from a group of people. You may have to appeal to each Brain Color individual to get everyone on board with an idea.
—Participant at an Advocate Condell Medical Center Leadership Development Program

For more information about Sheila's educational, entertaining, and engaging **What Color Is Your Brain?®** Programs for your health care professional development conference or meetings, contact Sheila by e-mail at **sheila@sheilaglazov.com** and visit her website at **www.sheilaglazov.com**.